Advance Praise for *The Great Health Dilemma*

It may seem self-evident that prevention is better than cure, but we seldom act as if we believed it. In this brilliant work, Christopher Dye describes the many ways prevention is undervalued in comparison to its demonstrable benefits. Everyone who cares about the public's health—and their own—has much to gain from absorbing Dye's lessons.

Harvey V. Fineberg, President,
Gordon and Betty Moore Foundation

In a chapter on unlikely disasters, Chris Dye explores pandemic preparedness as a highly topical example of prevention. Invoking principles used throughout the book, he argues that Covid-19 should be seen not as an isolated, once-in-a-lifetime event, but rather as one among hundreds of outbreaks of infectious diseases that are recorded each year. Borrowing ideas from the insurance industry, he suggests pooling all risks and sharing the costs to fund the development of generic "platform" technologies – precursors for diagnostics, therapeutics and vaccines that can be into called into action to combat a wide variety of pathogens as they emerge. This is a book for all who are concerned about the disruption of our planet, and about the increased opportunities that it creates for emergence of infectious pathogens at the animal/human interface.

David L. Heymann, Professor,
Infectious Disease Epidemiology,
London School of Hygiene and Tropical Medicine

By incisively dissecting the dialectical relationship between prevention and treatment of illness, Chris Dye has laid bare one of the great contradictions in health. His razor-sharp analysis unravels the complexity of our values and choices that has seen prevention remaining a poor neglected cousin of treatment. A truly enlightening book - a must-read!

Salim S. Abdool Karim,
CAPRISA Professor of Global Health,
Department of Epidemiology,
Mailman School of Public Health,
Columbia University

Using the example of TB, Chris Dye explains that by addressing the underlying risk factors and determinants for the disease, one would in fact be preventing a host of other health conditions and improving wellbeing. While biological and immunological reasons make finding a vaccine for TB challenging, we should also be addressing environmental, economic, and social risk factors for ill health.

Soumya Swaminathan,
Chief Scientist,
World Health Organization

T0177671

The Great Health Dilemma

Is Prevention Better than Cure?

Christopher Dye

Professor of Epidemiology, University of Oxford

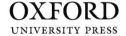

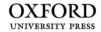

OXFORD
UNIVERSITY PRESS

Great Clarendon Street, Oxford, OX2 6DP,
United Kingdom

Oxford University Press is a department of the University of Oxford.
It furthers the University's objective of excellence in research, scholarship,
and education by publishing worldwide. Oxford is a registered trade mark of
Oxford University Press in the UK and in certain other countries

Impression: 1

First Edition published in 2021

Published in the United States of America by Oxford University Press
198 Madison Avenue, New York, NY 10016, United States of America

British Library Cataloguing in Publication Data

Data available

Library of Congress Control Number: 2020952931

ISBN 978–0–19–885382–4

DOI: 10.1093/oso/9780198853824.001.0001

Printed and bound by
CPI Group (UK) Ltd, Croydon, CR0 4YY

Preface

'If I were you, I wouldn't start from here.'
Directions allegedly given to a destination in Ireland.

The proverbial benefits of prevention over cure are, on the face of it, self-evident. A healthy life is one spent free of illness, and in full fitness, until the moment of death. That is surely better than struggling against acute, chronic, or recurrent bouts of sickness. Based on that sentiment, it is no surprise that the preference for prevention over cure has been expressed, in assorted ways, throughout human history.

But if prevention is so desirable why, paradoxically, do we invest so little in staying healthy and so much on curing illness?[1] The widely disseminated facts about spending on health in the world's wealthiest nations (members of the Organisation for Economic Co-operation and Development [OECD]) highlight the apparent inconsistency: just 3% of the US$6.8 trillion spent on health worldwide in 2017 was allocated to prevention and public health, while more than 90% was spent on treatment, rehabilitation, and long-term care.[2–4]

Health professionals argue that we should spend much more than 3% based on a large volume of economic analysis, which finds that prevention is often cost-effective and sometimes even cost-saving.[5–12] Part of the economic argument is that preventing illness helps to offset the rising costs of clinical treatments, which are forced upwards by new medical technologies, by market-driven pricing mechanisms for drugs and other medical commodities, by higher expectations linked to rising incomes, and by the growing healthcare needs of ageing populations.[13–15]

Across the European Union in 2015, around 570,000 deaths (out of 1.7 million deaths in people under 75 years) could have been avoided if healthcare systems had offered timely and effective medical treatments. But many more deaths—over a million—could have been avoided by better prevention and public health.[16]

The benefits of prevention come from avoiding hazards from the environment (such as polluted water and unsafe sanitation), from metabolic disorders (including diabetes and overweight), and from risky behaviours (especially alcohol and tobacco use, poor diet, and physical inactivity). In 2019, these risks accounted, respectively, for at least 20%, 33%, and 38% of all deaths worldwide.[17] These figures are in line with other assessments showing that social, economic, and environmental factors, in combination, typically explain 45%–60% of the variation in the health status of populations, as measured by life expectancy.[18-20] To the extent that these factors can be modified, they should be targets for preventing ill health.

Such facts about the preventable causes of illness and death, and many more like them, are frequently recited. Less thoroughly studied, with a few notable exceptions,[1,21,22] are the reasons why prevention is given low priority, and the possible remedies. The premise of this book—and its main testable proposition—is that decisions that disfavour prevention are not irrational 'false economies', as portrayed by some economic evaluations.[6,23-25] Rather, they are rational choices, considering the options on offer, the limits to resources, the threats to health, and the beliefs, motives, commitments, perceptions, and values of those who have the power to choose.[26-28] The pathway to better prevention comes, not from insisting that it is the right course of action, but from understanding why many people behave as if it is not, and why they might change their minds.

The paradox of disease prevention is actually the dilemma faced by any organism carrying any assets into an uncertain future. With regard to human behaviour, the 'dilemma' implies that we want to know, not merely that prevention and treatment are options, but what motives lead to the choice of one over the other. 'Rational' does not necessarily require conscious decision making by a selfish *Homo economicus* exercising free will ('Econs', as Richard Thaler called them). It suggests that the observed choices—the product of biological, behavioural, and cultural evolution—are made because they confer an advantage, and that they are susceptible to reasoned explanation, even if the reasons are not immediately obvious (at first sight 'irrational'). This is a book about humans rather than Econs.

In making a better case for investing in good health, unreasoned advocacy for safer and healthier lifestyles is generally unpersuasive. The rhetorical view, for instance, that *salus populi suprema lex* (public health must be the highest law) resonates mostly with those who already agree.[29] Instead of preaching to the converted, effort is better directed at convincing the dissenters—by understanding their values, powers, preferences, and motives. If, for example, health is a political choice, political leaders must have a reason for making that choice.[30]

Much is at stake. For the architects of the United Nations 2030 Agenda for Sustainable Development, prevention is an indispensable tool for surviving the twenty-first century. The Sustainable Development Goals (SDGs) make health central to human development, recognizing that good health depends on, and contributes to, other development goals, which underpin social justice, economic prosperity, and environmental protection.[31] Despite continued improvements in health and life expectancy since 2000, progress is currently too slow to meet most of the SDGs by 2030, including those for health.[32,33] Reaching these goals depends, not just on having access to essential health services, but also on finding long-term solutions to the root causes of ill health: chronic diseases of ageing populations, persistent poverty and hunger, poor education, income inequality, growing slum settlements, unsustainable agriculture, a pandemic of fast food consumption and obesity, polluting energy and transport, overexploited terrestrial and marine ecosystems, and climate change.

And yet medicine and public health, in richer and poorer countries alike, are still largely reactive instead of proactive—organized around the response to illness and injury rather than around the means of preserving and enhancing health. There is good reason for questioning that imbalance: if, in a rational world, the benefits of prevention were thought to exceed the costs—monetary and non-monetary, objective and subjective—then tens of millions of disease episodes could be averted each year.

This investigation of the health dilemma—is prevention better than cure?—begins by tracing the history of prevention over the past 5,000 years. Chapter 1, 'History of a hypothesis', shows that all the essential features of the age-old quandary are exposed under history's hugely varying circumstances. History makes no predictions, but it does offer insights that help to make decisions for the future. For all today's choices, though they are contemporary in detail and context, there is guidance in historical precedents.

Principles emerge from precedents: they help interpret the past and generate testable ideas about the future. Chapter 2, 'The problem of prevention', frames investment in health as insurance (or assurance) against the risk of future illness. The general, testable hypothesis driving this investigation is that insurance ought to be worth the premium when preventive methods can eliminate a large, imminent threat to health, with a high degree of certainty and at relatively low cost.

We can measure a threat to health, and the cost of removing that threat, and this is done routinely in economic evaluations. But every decision about health depends on the way values are assigned to facts, by everyone who has a stake—citizens, governments, non-governmental organizations, businesses and researchers, among others—each of whom may have different goals. Not even the agreed professional criteria for carrying out economic evaluations are free from subjectivity. In testing ideas about prevention, subjective values, as well as objective facts, set the conditions for evaluation.

Chapter 2 explains why, despite the enduring proverb, prevention is often less appealing than cure a priori. This sets up the challenge: to show how disadvantage can be turned to advantage by manipulating the incentives for action—the feasible choices, the reward for investment, and the certainty and immediacy with which the reward will be obtained. There are practical as well as conceptual challenges on the way: one of them is that public health guidance commonly states the desired endpoint—for instance, an affordable or cost-effective solution—without mapping out the route from origin to destination (thus the Irish joke at the head of the chapter).

Chapters 3–8 illustrate the challenges and how to confront them, with six main themes: competition for limited resources, the management of risk, the perception of hazard, the cultural and social context of health choices, and the present value of the future.

Chapter 3, 'The affordable dream', highlights prevention's disadvantage in competing for limited resources. From the perspective of government, prevention offers health benefits that lie within and outside the scope of health services. And yet prevention is a government orphan. When health is the primary purpose (as in government health departments), prevention cannot compete directly with clinical care; when health is a secondary benefit (agriculture, education, environment, and transport departments), prevention might influence the agenda but rarely has the casting vote.

Chapter 4, 'Unlikely disasters', focuses on the assessment and management of risk. The prevention of rare, unpredictable, diverse, high-impact disasters and emergencies, from earthquakes to Ebola, must balance the cost and efficacy of investment now against the likely risk, timing, and magnitude of a future disaster. Much of this book was written before the coronavirus pandemic broke late in 2019: COVID-19 has subsequently illustrated, not fundamentally changed, the principles of managing unlikely disasters.

Chapter 5, 'Normal ways to die', considers how health hazards are perceived and misperceived, as determinants of action. Major endemic infections, such as tuberculosis and HIV/AIDS, cause a persistently high burden of disease worldwide partly because the options for prevention are still limited, despite decades of research. While the numbers of deaths attributable to these two infections are large, the risk per person is low, familiar, and predictable, all factors that diminish the value of the threat, as perceived by the public and by public health services. Tuberculosis has probably killed more people than any other infection in history, but it is rarely considered a public health emergency like COVID-19, Ebola, or pandemic influenza.

Chapter 6, 'The burden of choice', asks who is able to choose, and who is responsible for choosing, between prevention and cure. Nowadays. most people die, not from infections, but from chronic, non-communicable diseases—heart disease, stroke, cancers, chronic lung disease, and diabetes—much of which can be prevented by tackling major 'risk factors', including alcohol and tobacco; sugar, salt, and saturated fat in food; and physical inactivity. Lessening exposure to these hazards is compromised by a dispute that is central to prevention—on the balance between individual and social responsibility for choice.[34]

Chapter 7, 'The culture of conveniences', puts prevention in cultural context. Sanitation is commonly viewed as an instrument of good health, but effective sanitation depends on aligning health goals with other interests, most of which are more important to users than health—personal toilet preferences; social norms of defecation; water and waste management at household and city scales; energy and food production; crop irrigation and animal husbandry. Sanitation represents the classic problem of how to improve health in the wider context of society, environment, and economy.

Chapter 8, 'Our children's children', is about elevating concern today for illness and injury that will happen in the discounted future. Climate change—prevention's greatest challenge—is a large and growing threat to health, and leads concern about the health effects of environmental degradation more generally.[35–38] But amid the deluge of bleak forecasts of climate change and its consequences, there is a more hopeful story: we appear to be on the cusp of a rapidly accelerating transition towards decarbonization through mitigation and adaptation.

Chapter 9, 'Future positive', concludes with 12 lessons for prevention, distilled from principle and practice. These are methods and motives for shifting the balance away from reactive medical treatment, bypassing illness and injury, on the road to WHO's 'state of complete physical, mental, and social well-being'.[39,40]

Behind the whole narrative is an ambition common to all science—to investigate how a diverse set of questions, demanding a broad range of answers, can be understood in terms of a few common principles. The practical suggestions on how to make the case for prevention are far from being the last word (Chapter 9). The arguments, the evidence, and the possibilities are simply an effort to help 'dispel the mist, and fix the outlines of the vague form which is looming through it'.[41]

References

1. Fineberg HV. The paradox of disease prevention: Celebrated in principle, resisted in practice. *Journal of the American Medical Association* 2013; *310*: 85–90.
2. Organisation for Economic Co-operation and Development (OECD), Eurostat, and World Health Organization. *A System of Health Accounts 2011: Revised Edition*. Paris: OECD; 2017.
3. Gmeinder M, Morgan D, Mueller M. *How Much Do OECD Countries Spend on Prevention?* Paris: OECD; 2017.
4. Office for National Statistics. UK health accounts: 2016. 2016. https://www.ons.gov.uk/peoplepopulationandcommunity/healthandsocialcare/healthcaresystem/bulletins/ukhealthaccounts/2016#total-healthcare-expenditure-by-function-and-provider (accessed 7 January 2021).
5. Hale J, Phillips CJ, Jewell T. Making the economic case for prevention—a view from Wales. *BMC Public Health* 2012; *12*: 460.
6. Masters R, Anwar E, Collins B, Cookson R, Capewell S. Return on investment of public health interventions: A systematic review. *Journal of Epidemiology & Community Health* 2017; *71*: 827–34.
7. Suhrcke M, Urban D, Moesgaard Iburg K, Schwappach D, Boluarte T, McKee M. *The Economic Benefits of Health and Prevention in a High-Income Country: The Example of Germany*. Berlin: Wissenschaftszentrum Berlin für Sozialforschung (WZB); 2007.
8. Owen L, Morgan A, Fischer A, Ellis S, Hoy A, Kelly MP. The cost-effectiveness of public health interventions. *Journal of Public Health (Oxford Academic)* 2012; *34*: 37–45.
9. van Gils PF, Tariq L, Verschuuren M, van den Berg M. Cost-effectiveness research on preventive interventions: A survey of the publications in 2008. *European Journal of Public Health* 2011; *21*: 260–4.
10. Owen L, Fischer A. The cost-effectiveness of public health interventions examined by the National Institute for Health and Care Excellence from 2005 to 2018. *Public Health* 2019; *169*: 151–62.
11. World Health Organization (WHO) Regional Office for Europe. *The Case for Investing in Public Health*. Copenhagen: WHO Regional Office for Europe; 2014.
12. British Medical Association. *Exploring the Cost Effectiveness of Early Intervention and Prevention*. London: British Medical Association; 2017.
13. Fuchs VR. How to make US health care more equitable and less costly: Begin by replacing employment-based insurance. *JAMA* 2018; *320*(20): 2071–2.

14. OECD. Healthcare costs unsustainable in advanced economies without reform. 2015. http://www.oecd.org/health/healthcarecostsunsustainableinadvancedec onomieswithoutreform.htm (accessed 7 January 2021).

15. Phelps C, Madhavan G. Patents and drug insurance: Clash of the titans? *Science Translational Medicine* 2018; *10*: 467.

16. Eurostat. Are 570,000 deaths per year in the EU avoidable? 2018. https:// ec.europa.eu/eurostat/web/products-eurostat-news/-/DDN-20180629-1 (accessed 7 January 2021).

17. Institute for Health Metrics and Evaluation (IHME). GBD Results Tool. 2020. http://ghdx.healthdata.org/gbd-results-tool (accessed 7 January 2021).

18. The King's Fund. Broader determinants of health: Future trends. 2020. https:// www.kingsfund.org.uk/projects/time-think-differently/trends-broader-determinants-health (accessed 7 January 2021).

19. Donkin A, Goldblatt P, Allen J, Nathanson V, Marmot M. Global action on the social determinants of health. *BMJ Global Health* 2018; *3*(Suppl. 1): e000603.

20. Webber L, Chalkidou K, Morrow S, Ferguson B, McPherson K. What are the best societal investments for improving people's health? *BMJ* 2018; *362*: k3377.

21. Russell LB. Is Prevention Better than Cure? Washington, DC: Brookings Institution; 1986.

22. McGinnis JM, Williams-Russo P, Knickman JR. The case for more active policy attention to health promotion. *Health Affairs (Millwood)* 2002; *21*: 78–93.

23. Ferguson B. Cost savings and the economic case for investing in public health. Public Health Matters, 9 April 2018, Public Health England.

24. Ferguson B. Investing in prevention: The need to make the case now. Public Health Matters, 22 February 2016, Public Health England.

25. Finch D. New reductions to the public health grant will heap more pressure on local authorities. 2018. www.health.org.uk/search/basic_page_sub_type/54 (accessed 7 January 2021).

26. Allin S, Mossialos E, McKee M, Holland W. *Making Decisions in Public Health: A Review of Eight Countries*. Copenhagen: World Health Organization; 2004.

27. Hauck K, Smith PC. Public choice analysis of public health priority setting. In: Culyer AJ, ed. *Encyclopedia of Health Economics*. San Diego, Elsevier; 2014: 184–93.

28. Sen A. Rational fools: A critique of the behavioral foundations of economic theory. *Philosophy & Public Affairs* 1977; *6*: 317–44.

29. Spinney L. How pandemics shape social evolution. *Nature* 2019; *574*: 324–6.

30. Kickbusch I, Kirton J. *Health: A Political Choice*. London: Global Governance Project, GT Media Group Ltd; 2020.

31. Dye C. Expanded health systems for sustainable development. *Science* 2018; *359*: 1337–9.

32. World Health Organization. *World Health Statistics 2020: Monitoring Health for the SDGs, Sustainable Development Goals*. Geneva: WHO; 2020.

33. United Nations. *The Sustainable Development Goals Report 2020*. New York: United Nations; 2020.

34. Wanless D. *Securing Good Health for the Whole Population*. London: Her Majesty's Stationery Office; 2004.

35. Guterres A. Secretary-General's remarks on climate change. 2018. https://www. un.org/sg/en/content/sg/statement/2018-09-10/secretary-generals-remarks-climate-change-delivered (accessed 7 January 2021).

36. European Academies Science Advisory Council. *The Imperative of Climate Action to Protect Human Health in Europe.* Halle: German National Academy of Sciences Leopoldina; 2019.

37. Marzouk S, Choi H. *What Does the Next 25 Years Hold for Global Health?* London: Royal Society of Tropical Medicine and Hygiene; 2019.

38. Watts N, Amann M, Ayeb-Karlsson S, et al. The Lancet Countdown on health and climate change: from 25 years of inaction to a global transformation for public health. *Lancet* 2018; 391: 581–630.

39. World Health Organization. *Constitution.* Geneva: WHO; 1948.

40. OECD. Measuring well-being and progress: Well-being research. 2019. https:// www.oecd.org/statistics/measuring-well-being-and-progress.htm. (accessed 7 January 2021).

41. Mill JS. Bentham. In: Robson JM, ed. *The Collected Works of John Stuart Mill, Volume X—Essays on Ethics, Religion, and Society.* London: Routledge and Kegan Paul; 1985.

Acknowledgements

Is prevention really better than cure? That question has been present throughout the 40 years I have worked in universities and public health agencies, especially the World Health Organization (WHO). Having left WHO in 2018, my own ideas about how to answer it have taken clearer form in various parts of Europe, from the Amsterdam Stadhuis (seventeenth-century organization of public services) to the sewers of Paris (nineteenth-century revolution in public health) to locked down Oxford (twenty-first century response to the COVID-19 pandemic). I began writing this book at All Souls College, Oxford, in 2018 and (nearly) finished it at the Oxford Martin School in 2020. I am enormously grateful to John Vickers and Charles Godfray, the heads of those two institutions, for giving me the time and space to work there, and to Angela McLean who helped organize both.

COVID-19 scuppered deadlines but had the benefit of testing some of the ideas already discussed with colleagues and friends. Those who helped me, wittingly or unwittingly, in agreement or disagreement, include Jo Bibby, Enricke Bouma, Sandy Cairncross, Ted Cohen, Paul Coleman, Vince Crawford, John Crump, Andy Dobson, Christl Donnelly, Michael Fraser, Charles Godfray, Shaun Hargreaves-Heap, Katharina Hauck, Cameron Hepburn, David Heymann, Guy Hutton, Susan Jebb, Alex Kacelnik, Frank Kelly, Joe Kutzin, Tim Lenton, Jim Malcomson, Anne Mills, Michael Mueller, David Parkin, Lucia Prauscello, Lant Pritchett, Jennifer Rampling, Jeffrey Stanaway, Brian Williams, Tom Williams, Andrew Wilson, and Ke Xu. The mistakes are mine; when they are discovered, I shall lean on James Thurber ('Don't get it right, get it written').

Two people at Oxford University Press did help get it written. Nicola Wilson gave me sound advice from the start, and Rachel Goldsworthy guided the project in its closing stages. Both remained patient during the COVID-induced delay—before I finally got to The End.

Contents

Abbreviations

AIDS	acquired immune deficiency syndrome
AMR	antimicrobial or antibiotic resistance
ART	antiretroviral therapy
BCG	Bacillus Calmette–Guérin
CEPI	Coalition for Epidemic Preparedness Innovations
CLTS	Community-led total sanitation
COPD	chronic obstructive pulmonary disease
COVID-19	coronavirus disease
DALY	disability-adjusted life year
DIB	Development Impact Bond
DOTS	directly observed treatment, short course
ETEC	enterotoxigenic *Escherichia coli*
FFV	flex-fuel vehicle
GAVI	Global Alliance on Vaccines and Immunization
GDP	gross domestic product
GISAID	Global Initiative on Sharing Avian Influenza Data
GWP	Global warming potential
GRID	gay-related immune deficiency syndrome
GVP	Global Virome Project
HCM	healthy condition monitoring
HiAP	health in all policies
HIV	human immunodeficiency virus
IARC	International Agency for Research on Cancer
IDSR	Integrated Disease Surveillance and Response
IHR	International Health Regulations
LPG	Liquefied petroleum gas
LRI	lower respiratory infection
MERS	Middle East respiratory syndrome
MDG	Millennium Development Goal
NTD	neglected tropical disease
NGO	non-governmental organization
NICE	National Institute for Health and Care Excellence
NIPH	National Institute for Health Protection
OECD	Organisation for Economic Co-operation and Development
O&M	Operations and maintenance

OR	operational research
ORT	oral rehydration therapy
PEF	Pandemic Emerging Finance Facility
PIP	Pandemic Influenza Preparedness
PCP	Pneumocystis carinii pneumonia
PreP	pre-exposure prophylaxis
PHEIC	Public Health Emergency of International Concern
QALY	quality-adjusted life year
R&D	research and development
RITE	Rapid Isolation and Treatment of Ebola
SARS	severe acute respiratory syndrome
SCLP	short-lived climate pollutant
SHA	System of Health Accounts
SIB	Social Impact Bond
SDG	Sustainable Development Goal
SDI	socio-demographic index
TB	tuberculosis
UNICEF	United Nations Children's Fund
UNMEER	United Nations Mission for the Emergency Ebola Response
UHC	Universal Health Coverage
WASH	water, sanitation, and hygiene
WHO	World Health Organization

1
History of a hypothesis

> The skillful doctor treats those who are well, the inferior doctor treats those who are ill.
>
> Pien Ch'iao, Chinese surgeon (third century BC)

A proverb's short-cut to wisdom often conceals a more circuitous route to the truth. To understand how we see the future today, it is worth looking at how we saw it in the past. Running over millennia, the recorded human history of disease prevention is a tale of hope and expectation, risk and uncertainty, truth and perception, science and superstition, power and control, individual and collective action, and of the valued present (*carpe diem*) versus the devalued future (*mañana*). The account given here, like most others, is biased towards the well-documented (in English) western world. Its purpose, however, is not to be comprehensive or categorical; rather, it is to suggest that the main ideas about prevention have a long pedigree even if, in every age and in every place, they find new interpretation.

On the preservation of health

For all biological organisms, reproductive success is measured by the number of offspring produced in the next generation. Success depends on maximizing this reproductive number in the face of adversity—including disease, injury, and death. In principle, more offspring might be produced by investing in prevention rather than treatment and cure. If the mechanism of prevention is heritable, transmissible from parent to offspring through the genome, then it would be subject to evolution by natural selection. Alternatively, or in addition, a successful preventive behaviour, once

The Great Health Dilemma. Christopher Dye, Oxford University Press. © Oxford University Press 2021.
DOI: 10.1093/oso/9780198853824.003.0001

discovered, can be learned and memorized by others, spreading through a population as a form of cultural evolution.

There are abundant examples of prevention throughout the animal kingdom (putting aside other forms of life). Animals can anticipate the future using a mix of genetic and cultural evolution, as illustrated by behaviours that favour prevention over cure in self- and group-medicating species.[1,2] European wood ants, *Formica paralugubris*, use conifer resin to prevent bacterial and fungal infections in their nests.[3,4] Venezuelan capuchin monkeys rub millipede secretions containing insect repellent benzoquinones into their fur during the wet season peak in biting insect abundance.[5] Both are examples of prophylactic rather than therapeutic treatment in animals where prevention has been favoured as an alternative or as a complement to cure. Such observations on primates suggest that behaviours which preserve health and prevent disease have a long evolutionary and cultural history in their human descendants, spanning hundreds of thousands of years.

On that timescale, the first inferences about human preventive behaviour are relatively recent. Eating, drinking, washing, and defecating have always been essential for life; nutritious food, clean water, and safe sanitation are vital for the preservation of health and the prevention of disease.[6] The first efforts to manage the distribution of water—with dams and irrigation systems—were driven by the need to produce enough food to live in the Tigris and Euphrates (Mesopotamia, *c*.5300 BC), Nile (*c*.3300 BC) and Indus (*c*.2800 BC) river valleys. Irrigation for agriculture was the precursor to urban water and sanitation systems as small and scattered farming villages grew into conurbations, making greater demands to cooperate in providing food and water supplies and on waste management in increasingly dense, sedentary populations.[7]

Based on archaeological evidence from the third millennium BC, the Neolithic peoples of Central America (Guatemala), Europe (Orkney Islands), Mediterranean (Crete), the Middle East (Israel, Turkey), North Africa (Egypt), and South Asia (Indus valley) had the means and motives to filter and boil water, to design and build flushable cesspits and toilets, and communal drains and sewerage systems.[8] The great variety of efforts to purify water, and to remove excreta and other waste, suggest that the environmental causes of illness were understood, and understood to be preventable, with health benefits for individuals and whole communities.[9,10]

By the third millennium BC (if not before), physicians were carrying out surgery and had accumulated a rich pharmacopeia of medicinal plants and minerals for healing. The Egyptian practice of applying a poultice of mouldy bread to an infected wound might be the first instance of antibiotic treatment. More than this, and in spite of the prevailing causal model of disease as divine punishment (penitence was cure, not prevention), doctors also gave advice on staying healthy—for instance, by washing and shaving the body to prevent conditions now known to be caused by infections.[11] There were treatments for patients and penitents; and, for some conditions at least, there were means of prevention too.

From the sixth century BC onwards, Greek philosophy sharpened the distinction between natural science and theology in pursuit of a reasoned understanding of causes and effects. Knowing the cause is a precondition for reliably preventing the effect. Health and disease were known to be associated with the physical and social environments in which people lived, and with human behaviour.[12,13] Hippocrates' (c.460–375 BC) *On Airs, Waters and Places* (c.400 BC) was a guide to preventing illness for settlers in new environments.[14] Some of the advice was common sense: houses should be built in elevated and sunny areas, avoiding marshes and malarial swamps. Some drew on prevailing aetiological theory: dietary regimens and regular exercise could maintain 'a healthy mind in a healthy body', ostensibly by keeping in balance the four humours—black bile, yellow bile, phlegm, and blood.[15] These ideas are most frequently associated with Greece, but actually co-evolved across the ancient civilized world: during the first millennium BC, humoral balance was integral to physiological models of health in contemporary Hindu (Ayurveda) and Chinese societies too.

Prevention was taken seriously by Greek physicians. According to Pliny the Elder (23–79 AD), Asclepiades of Bithynia (c.124–40 BC) staked his medical reputation on prevention by making a bet with [the goddess] Fortune 'that he should not be considered a doctor if ever he himself fell ill in any way'.[16] He is said to have died by falling down stairs, aged 84, thus escaping the ignominy of terminal illness, winning his bet posthumously and securing his legacy in preventive medicine.

However, prevention went far beyond the practice of physicians. Underpinning medicine, Greek democracy was an instrument of public health. Individuals and communities were empowered through participatory institutions, emphasizing education and the development of skills to maintain good health. This was 'health promotion'—enabling people to increase control over and improve their health—two thousand years before its rebranding in the twentieth century.[13] It perhaps illustrated, too, the scale on which enabling must take place if health promotion is to succeed (Chapter 8).

Ever since people began to live in settled communities, they have been forced to relieve themselves of bodily waste, not just personally, but as whole populations. Driven by this sanitary imperative, private and communal toilets linked to drains and sewers became common from at least the third millennium BC. Between 500 BC and 500 AD, public water supply and sewage systems, albeit imperfect systems, were hallmarks of Greece and Rome.

In antiquity, risk was often seen in terms of fate and met with acceptance rather than defiance.[17] But not always: pragmatic traders—Babylonian, Chinese, Greek, and Indian, from the second millennium BC onwards—not content with the hand of fortune, also understood how to invest in prevention in the face of uncertainty and adversity.

Their understanding created foundations for the insurance industry. Risk is non-fungible, or non-transferable, for individuals. But risk can be shared among individuals in a group. So individuals exposed to losses through common risks naturally grouped together in order to aggregate the risk, put a price on it, and sell it to investors (Chapter 4).[18] Insurance is an instrument of prevention as well as cure.

For shipping, risk was not necessarily mitigated by financial compensation for loss. It was often non-financial and preventive—for example, by steering clear of sea passages known to be dangerous (which required collaboration through record keeping and the exchange of information), by arming ships as a deterrent to pirates, and by spreading risk by dividing a cargo among several vessels.

In maritime trading, 'bottomry' contracts provided loans to shipping merchants, secured on the bottom or keel of a ship. When the ship returned to port after a voyage, the loan was repaid with interest. If the shipment was lost at sea, the loan was forfeited by the guarantor. This form of insurance, in which the chance of gain and risk of loss are transferred from merchant to investor, resembles a modern catastrophe bond. It provides guarantors with incentives for prevention—invest in safe ships. Whether the idea of insurance was also applied to the risk of illness in antiquity is apparently unknown, but catastrophe bonds are one of the instruments used nowadays to protect health and life from hurricanes, epidemics, and other disasters (Chapter 4).

Some of the wisdom of Ancient Greece found continuity in Classical Rome, as recorded in practice and proverb. Galen (129–*c*.210 AD), 'first among doctors' in the opinion of Emperor Marcus Aurelius, was renowned for his discoveries in anatomy and physiology to inform medical treatments. But he also taught that a physician's priority was to keep people in good health. Galen's physiological model of good health expanded the Greek theory of balancing humours by regulating the 'non-naturals' (as Arab scholars later called them). The non-naturals or necessities to be regulated were air, food and drink, sleep and wakefulness, motion and rest, evacuation and repletion, and the passions of the mind, with occasional add-ons including baths, exercise, and sex.[19]

Galen believed in good health and well-being for all, founded not merely on philosophy and medicine but also on the physical constructs of urban life: gymnasia, aqueducts, bath houses and communal toilets, streets and public meeting places. His *Hygiene* (or *On the Preservation of Health*) identified education as vital to learning what was harmful and what was beneficial for health. To the extent that the theory and its practice were beneficial, they did not significantly lengthen life expectancy, which in the Roman Empire was typically 20–30 years from birth. Military campaigns carried an obvious risk of disease and injury for adult males, but death rates were far higher in children under five years old.[20] Nevertheless, Galen's synthesis of medical practice in general, and of prevention in particular, had wide appeal and astonishing longevity—influencing health and medicine globally for more than a thousand years.

Greco–Roman progress in science and medicine slowed in Europe with the decline of the western Roman empire from the fourth century AD but continued to flourish in the east. Roman and Byzantine Constantinople became a centre for experimentation and empirical observation. Constantinople, situated at the junction between Europe and Asia, also served as a conduit for Greek and Roman thought into the Islamic world where it developed through cross-fertilization with Indian and Persian medicine.

The Islamic Golden Age (*c*.750–1258) produced a succession of polymaths who expanded the concepts and methods of disease prevention and treatment. An array of Arabic medical texts offered technical solutions for environmental pollution and the management of municipal waste. Rhazes (854–925) studied the effects of diet, hygiene, climate, and seasonality on health. Avicenna's (980–1037) encyclopaedic *Canon of Medicine* (1025), published at the turn of the first millennium, synthesized more than a thousand years of medical practice from the Egyptian, Greek, Roman, Indian, Christian, Jewish, and Islamic worlds. The *Canon* was as much a treatise on prevention as on cure, for the dual 'goal of medicine is keeping health and returning it while having disease'.[21]

That which preserveth health is more excellent

Mediaeval Christian Europe (500–1000), maligned as the Dark Ages, was not so dark as commonly portrayed. Instances of scientific censorship in the Middle Ages were outnumbered by examples of the Roman Catholic Church acting as custodian, funder, and promoter of mediaeval intellectual advancement. This was neither doctrinally inconsistent nor scientifically prejudicial: as Aristotle (384–322 BC) had concluded much earlier, if the natural world was governed by God's laws, then studying nature would be one way to understand His purpose. Gaining that understanding may not have been motivated by an earthly need for innovation, but it certainly permitted it. Mediaeval agriculture, for example, was a beneficiary: productivity increased with the development of heavy ploughs, crop rotation, and watermills. Besides, the Church's mission was also to serve the needs of the poor, and the remedies for poverty were secular as well as spiritual.

In terms of public health in Europe, the Middle Ages were bracketed by two major pandemics of plague (later known to be caused by the flea-borne bacterium, *Yersinia pestis*)—the Plague of Justinian in 542 and the Black Death in 1348, with frequent smaller outbreaks in between. The high burden of sickness and death caused by plague, leprosy, and other contagious diseases was a powerful impetus to seek pragmatic solutions. There was no medical cure for plague so the best tactic was prevention: known or suspected cases, and people who had been in contact with them, were isolated (e.g. for 40 days, 'quarantine') to stop the spread of disease.

Plague and leprosy were not the only targets for disease control. Motivated by the need to curb contagion more generally, public officials created a system of sanitary controls, using surveillance stations, isolation hospitals, and disinfection procedures. Efforts to improve sanitation included the development of pure water supplies, garbage and sewage disposal, and food inspection. Before national public health services were created, the value of personal and public hygiene was understood, if not diligently practised, by citizens and by local authorities alike.

From the early Middle Ages onwards, Latin and Greek translations of Islamic medical texts, including Avicenna's *Canon*, began to appear in

Europe. In this convergence of western and eastern thought, the idea of prevention resurfaced—for instance, in Henry de Bracton's *On the Laws and Customs of England* (*c*.1240). Once again, we read that 'it is better and more useful to meet a problem in time than to seek a remedy after the damage is done'.

Despite the advances made in the millennium since Galen, the task of the physician was still to maintain health by regulating the non-naturals, keeping the body in good 'temperament' and with an optimal 'complexion'.[22] Some facets of fourteenth-century health care were decidedly modern, such as attending to the particular requirements of each patient. Because complexion was known to differ among individuals, a satisfactory health regime would have to be tailored to individual needs, at least for those who could afford them. Thus, twenty-first century personalized or precision medicine, as it is now called, has a history of at least 700 years. Furthermore, the concept of prevention was applied to groups of people as well as to individual patients. Among these public health initiatives, regular prophylactic venesection (blood-letting) was prescribed for entire monastic communities, and healthy regimens were suggested for defined categories of vulnerable people—children or the elderly, or those living in unhealthy environments.

As the western world emerged from the Middle Ages, Galen's legacy was subjected to increasingly critical examination. Roger Bacon's (*c*.1219–92) *Greater Work* (*Opus Maius*), for instance, challenged conventional medical theories with experimental science. Doctors, he argued (after Horace), should take nothing on authority, specifically church authority; they should instead do their own empirical research.

Whether or not Bacon's advice was followed, the view that prevention trumps cure travelled more or less unscathed through the European Renaissance. Erasmus of Rotterdam (1466–1536), humanist scholar of classical antiquity (who was inclined to overlook advances made in the Middle Ages), reinforced the notion in his book of proverbs (the *Adages*) first published in 1500.[23] He is credited with stating that prevention is better than cure but he did not actually go that far. A more accurate translation of his Latin text is: 'It is better to treat at the beginning of illness than at the end' (*Adage* 1.ii.40). This falls short of true (primary) prevention because the emphasis is on the early diagnosis and treatment of illness, not on removing the underlying cause.

Other contemporary writers did promote strict prevention. One of them was Thomas Cogan who, echoing Avicenna's *Canon*, wrote in 1612: 'The art of Physicke hath two principall parts; the one declaring the order how health may be preserved: the other setting forth the meanes how sicknesse may bee remedied. Of these two parts that is more excellent which preserveth health and preventeth sicknesse.'[15,24]

An ounce of prevention

Prevention is better than cure, but not at any price. This insightful qualification was perhaps first made explicit in Benjamin Franklin's 'an ounce of prevention is worth a pound of cure' (1736), which has been widely generalized from his investigation of fire safety in Philadelphia. Because the costs of early versus late intervention are now quantified, at least metaphorically, this rendition of the proverb turns conventional wisdom into a conditional hypothesis. It is pedantic, of course, to ask whether the cost–benefit ratio is actually 1:16 (ounces in a pound); but it is sensible to ask, in general, whether benefits exceed costs, and under what circumstances.

Franklin's application to fire insurance had a long pedigree. The idea of insuring against risk had been in practical use for millennia (e.g. bottomry contracts already mentioned), including ways of insuring against fire. In AD 67, Nero had allegedly fiddled while Rome burned. He may well have dithered during the conflagration, but he undertook a costly rebuilding of the city thereafter, driven by imperial vanity but guided by, among other practicalities, fire precautions. According to Tacitus, 'from the ashes of the fire rose ... a city made of marble and stone with wide streets ... and ample supplies of water to quell any future blaze'.[25] New houses had to be built with fire walls, Rome acquired a fire department, and debris from the fire was used to fill nearby malarial swamps.

A century before Franklin, John Winthrop, Governor of Boston, Massachusetts, had in 1631 outlawed the building of homes with wooden chimneys and thatched roofs, which were recognized fire hazards. In Great Britain, the fire insurance industry was given a boost by the Great Fire of London in 1666. In the aftermath of the fire, the Rebuilding Act of 1667 was designed to prevent future disasters. Among other safety features, it required houses to have brick fronts, to be of equal height, and to have signs fixed to a wall rather than hanging over the street. Buildings had to be registered with city authorities and were checked against regulations by city surveyors.

Franklin's contribution in the 1750s was to set up one of America's first voluntary fire services (the Union Fire Company, also known as 'the Bucket Brigade'). But he also realized that, if fire is inevitable, and the timing and identity of victims are unpredictable, then it should be possible to set a premium for safety, affordable for everyone, based on the pooling of risk. He therefore established in 1751 the first colonial insurance company, the *Philadelphia Contributorship for the Insurance of Houses from Loss by Fire*. The *Contributorship* put a price on prudence, offering mutual insurance plans, 'whereby every man might help another, without any disservice to himself'. In gambling against ill fortune, this was a triple win: insurance gave peace of mind in the face of a fire risk, and of course it provided financial compensation for losses in the event of fire. But it also encouraged prevention: by inspecting properties to be insured, by setting premiums based on risk assessment, and by rejecting buildings that were not constructed to specified standards.

The categorical 'a stitch in time saves nine', attributed to astronomer Francis Baily (1797), also set costs against benefits. In fact, the original, less confident version is better: 'a stitch in time *may* save nine' properly captures the uncertainty associated with investing in the future. Like Erasmus' *Adages*, this form of the proverb calls for early diagnosis of an existing problem, rather than true prevention (no stitch needed at all). These different shades of proverbial wisdom highlight the question, still relevant today, of whether to invest in prevention proper (primary prevention), or to make do with early diagnosis (secondary prevention). The answer to the question depends on the costs and benefits of each strategy.

The eighteenth-century growth of experimental medicine led to improvements in the means of prevention, as well as creating better treatments. John Pringle's *Observations on the Diseases of the Army* (1752) spoke to problems of hospital ventilation and camp sanitation by advancing rules for proper drainage and latrines, and the avoidance of marshes. He insisted on sanitary measures that reduced the rate of typhus and dysentery, diseases that killed more soldiers than military conflict.

James Lind's *Treatise on the Scurvy* (1754) described his discovery that lemon juice prevented this severe skin and skeletal disease among British sailors (lime juice works too, hence 'limeys'). He did not need to know that scurvy was caused by vitamin C deficiency (vitamins were not discovered until 1912 and vitamin C not until 1928). He just needed to be able to design, carry out, and interpret his prototype of the controlled clinical trial.

Lind's study had its roots in the early seventeenth century. In 1601, Captain James Lancaster gave lemon juice to sailors on four ships, but not on another three 'control' ships. All the crew of the first four ships stayed healthy, whereas 110 of 278 men died of scurvy on the other three. In 1747, Lind extended the experiment by giving citrus fruits to scurvy patients who were cured in a few days. The British Navy adopted the policy in 1795 and eliminated scurvy entirely. In 1865, the British Board of Trade did the same for the merchant navy, with the same results. The time from discovery to full implementation in merchant and defence navies was 264 years.[26]

Variolation, the inoculation with smallpox virus to protect against severe disease later in life, was used in China from around 1000 AD. But it was Mary Wortley Montagu (1689–1762) who in 1721 famously introduced variolation to the western world.[27] She had observed the practice and its prophylactic power in Ottoman Turkey. Variolation clearly carried the risk of causing a severe episode of smallpox (with approximately a 2% chance of death), but Montagu nevertheless had her son (in Constantinople) and daughter (in England) inoculated. In August 1721, seven prisoners awaiting execution at Newgate Prison made their own calculation of risk when offered the chance to undergo variolation instead of execution. All were inoculated, all survived, and all were released.[28] The way they eventually died is not known, but it was probably not from smallpox. Setting the certainty of hindsight against the uncertainty of foresight, Benjamin Franklin greatly regretted that he had not made the same calculation on behalf of his own son. Four-year-old Francis Franklin died of smallpox in Boston in 1736 when inoculation was, on balance, probably worth the risk.[29]

After investigations in the 1760s and 1770s by physicians in England and Germany, in 1796, Edward Jenner 'vaccinated' an eight-year-old boy with pus from the hand of a milkmaid infected with the related cowpox virus (*vacca*, the cow). Jenner then boldly demonstrated that the boy was immune to challenge with smallpox infection. Farmers knew from practical experience that a mild episode of cowpox was protective against smallpox, but Jenner made the point experimentally and almost incontrovertibly (his study design would not satisfy modern standards of inference or ethics).

The road from smallpox variolation to vaccination is well known in the history of prevention. But variolation was not the only form of immunization with a long tradition. Cutaneous leishmaniasis is a skin disease caused by protozoan parasites in the genus *Leishmania* and transmitted by bloodsucking phlebotomine sandflies. Familiar in antiquity from North Africa across the Middle East to India, leishmanial lesions were variously known, with their geographical identifiers, as buttons (Basra), boils (Aleppo, Baghdad, Delhi, Jericho) and sores (Balkh, Oriental). For centuries, Bedouin, Kurdistani, and other tribal societies had practised leishmanization, the deliberate exposure of children to the parasite by the bite of a sandfly or the inoculation of infectious exudate from an active skin lesion. As with variolation, the aim was to produce a self-healing sore, which would be followed by long-lasting immunity. Immunity would protect against later disfiguring lesions on the face and other exposed parts of the body, especially crucial for the marriage prospects of a young woman.[30]

These advances in the scientific understanding of prevention, from lime juice to vaccination, needed a favourable medical, social, economic, and political environment for their application. Like anyone offering the next big idea, Pringle, Lind, Jenner, and other eighteenth-century pioneers had to overcome the scientific scepticism of their peers, plus the predictable opposition of those with vested interests, such as doctors making money out of risky variolation rather than the safer alternative, vaccination.

But there were larger societal forces at work. Through a succession of social revolutions between 1775 (America) and 1848 (Europe), these forces would help to create a more favourable environment for public health. In revolutionary late eighteenth-century Europe and America, the fortunate few in authority faced mounting pressure from the discontented many living in feudal poverty. In America, Thomas Jefferson (1743–1826) put health in context: in his view, despotism produced disease and democracy liberated health.[31] Out of the French revolution (1789–99) emerged the belief that healthy citizenship was a human right. And Europe's democratic advances leading up to the revolutions of 1848 provided the backdrop to advances in public health: medical police (Central Europe), statistical analysis of mortality (France), poor relief (Scotland), the provision of infirmaries (Ireland), and sanitation (England and Wales).[32]

Preventive police and the sanitary idea

In nineteenth-century Europe, the use of the word 'sanitation' made it clear that water and sewage were viewed as principal determinants of health and hygiene, even though citizens were more concerned then, as they are today, about privacy, comfort, odour, and the physical removal of urine and faeces (Chapter 7).[33,34] Unearthing the remnants of historical sanitation systems has drawn attention to the technology, but the implications for social organization are at least as important: advances in sanitation were products of early Indus valley culture, Greek democracy, Roman administration, and European Enlightenment humanitarianism.

Consequent to the latter, the huge increase in life expectancy enjoyed by people in the industrialized world since the eighteenth century is among the most remarkable biological events in human history.[35] No one living in Europe in the 1700s could have foreseen that life expectancy would increase so rapidly above the centuries-long norm of 20–40 years, more than doubling within two centuries. Within the changing social environment, the factors that lay behind the increase were cleaner water, safer sanitation, a more reliable supply of high-quality food, and a revolution in microbiology. Technological advances were coupled with accelerating economic growth, suggesting (but not proving) that there were mutually reinforcing, positive feedbacks between processes affecting health and the economy (Figure 1.1).

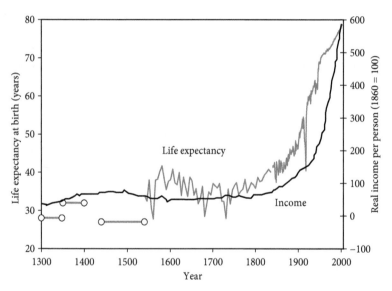

Figure 1.1 Up to 1800, life expectancy from birth in England and Wales was under 40 years (grey lines) but it more than doubled between 1800 and 2000. Income per person (black line) also accelerated sharply after 1800, suggesting that there was positive feedback between processes affecting health and the economy, although a third factor could have contributed to both.

Adapted with permission from Dye, C. (2010). 200 years in the history of longevity. *The Biologist*. 57 (3): 127–30.

The rise in life expectancy, driven mainly by the prevention of childhood infectious diseases, began a worldwide epidemiological and demographic transition. As a higher proportion of children survive to adulthood, parents choose to have smaller families. As infectious diseases wane, they are replaced by the chronic, non-communicable diseases typical of adulthood in larger, older populations. In Europe, North America, and other parts of the industrialized world, this transition took place over centuries. In some low- and middle-income countries, large reductions in mortality and fertility have taken place over just a few decades.[36]

The nineteenth-century sanitation 'revolution' was so-called, not because it was quick (it spanned the long life of Queen Victoria, 1819–1901) but because it was a national engineering project with effects that were ultimately enormous.

In England, Edwin Chadwick (1800–90), more than anyone else, put health in the broader social, economic, and environmental context. Passionate about state intervention for social good, Chadwick has been called the founder of English public health, though he and his collaborators, notably Thomas Southwood Smith, were products of the prevailing, and for them enabling, humanitarian outlook.[31] Elsewhere in Europe, others such as Rudolph Virchow (1821–1902) also championed the cause.

Chadwick pursued his mission partly through his role as a junior member of the Poor Law Commission of 1832. He became the main architect of the new Poor Law of 1834. The principle of the law was to make the conditions under which public relief could be given so unpleasant that most would refuse to request it. Popular objections to the law were understandable; as its administrator, Chadwick was said to be the most hated man in England.[32]

And yet his efforts delivered many benefits: the Commission stipulated that children should not work more than six hours a day and that employers should be held responsible for accidents in the workplace.[37] The work of the Poor Law Commission was followed by the Registration Act of 1836, which launched a public vaccination service in England. Under the first Vaccination Act, smallpox vaccination (replacing risky variolation) was at first optional (1840) and later made compulsory (1853).

But Chadwick's focus was on sanitation and what it could achieve. The stench of ordure and refuse was not new; it had long been a scourge of urban life in Europe,[38] but Chadwick skilfully advanced the case for hygiene in the face of complex sanitary politics. *The Means of Insurance against Accidents* (1828) developed his 'sanitary idea' for nationwide improvements to water supply and waste removal. His 1829 paper on 'Preventive Police' was an enquiry into 'the removable antecedents of crime'. This was a justification of state-controlled social welfare,[31] and a forerunner to Henry Rumsey's (1809–76) *Essays on State Medicine* (1856), which was, in effect, a practical guide for interventionists and preventionists: investigation, regulation, and prosecution carried out by the medical police.[39–41] Chadwick's crowning glory was his magisterial three-volume, systematic geographical study of health as a basis for action, the *Report on The Sanitary Condition of the Labouring Population of Great Britain* (1842).[8] The aims and methods of the *Report* were informed by, and in turn influenced, similar analyses in France and America, such as the sanitary reports for New York and Massachusetts, published, respectively, in 1845 and 1850.

The 1838 report of the Poor Law Commission promoted, once again, the view that prevention is better than cure: 'the expenditures necessary to the adoption and maintenance of measures of prevention would ultimately amount to less than the cost of the disease now constantly engendered'.[8] Inspired by Jeremy Bentham's (1748–1832) utilitarian ('felicific') calculus, Chadwick estimated 'that this expense [incurred by manual removal of decomposing refuse] may be reduced to one-twentieth or to one-thirtieth, or rendered inconsiderable, by the use of water and self-acting means of removal by improved and cheaper sewers and drains'. He went on to calculate, in an analysis of the kind still done today, 'that by the combinations of all these arrangements, it is probable that the full ensurable period of life, an increase of 13 years at least, may be extended to the whole of the labouring classes'.[42] Thirteen years was a big increase; retrospectively, that estimate looks justified by the remarkable growth in life expectancy (Figure 1.1).

The ensuing Public Health Act of 1848 was the first occasion on which a British government took national responsibility for the health of its citizens. Taking responsibility in this way inevitably provoked debate about whether preventive policing was in the public interest or an infringement of personal liberty. Sanitary engineering for better health was popular; sanitation as an instrument of social engineering much less so. The indomitable Chadwick personified the division of opinion. To enthusiasts, he was a pioneer of social reform; to dissenters, he was an agent of political oppression.[31,43]

In parallel with the 1848 Public Health Act, London's Metropolitan Sewer Commission (1848) made household sewer connections compulsory—relieving houses of the reek of cesspits but transferring the problem of pollution to the River Thames. The transition from cesspits to open sewers and faecally polluted rivers played out in different ways across Europe.[38] To remedy the Great Stink emanating from the Thames, the 1852 Metropolis (London) Water Act required all private water companies to move their intakes upstream and to install mechanisms for filtration. In fact, the private water companies were already investing in filtration systems to purify their water supplies, though they acted with varying speed and efficiency. That variation between water companies allowed physician John Snow (1813–58) to test his theory that cholera was caused by a water-borne infection rather than an air-borne miasma. During the first seven weeks of London's 1854 epidemic, Snow found that the number of cholera cases per capita was about eightfold higher in districts supplied by the Southwark and Vauxhall Water Company (intake downstream, poor filtration) as compared with those supplied by the Lambeth Waterworks Company (intake upstream, improved filtration).[44,45]

As part of the effort to curtail a cholera outbreak in the Golden Square district of London during 1854, Snow famously removed the handle of the Broad Street pump which, it was later discovered, dispensed water contaminated with the faeces of a choleric infant. Handles had previously been removed from pumps during cholera outbreaks in the United States. Snow's action in Broad Street actually had no discernible effect on the Golden Square outbreak, which was already in decline. But it was powerfully symbolic of a general truth about cholera: it is a water-borne disease.[45] Indeed, disabling the pump was just one of several precautions taken against cholera (liming of the streets was another) because local authorities remained unconvinced of Snow's argument. The eminent physician William Farr (1807–83) was not convinced until 1866. And, despite the Public Health Act of 1875, sewage pollution of the Thames continued until the 1880s. Definitive proof of the cause of cholera awaited experimental microbiology.

Preventive microbiology

Anton van Leeuwenhoek (1632–1723) had seen 'animalcules', including bacteria, through his new microscope in the 1670s but microbiology did not start to benefit from microscopy for another two centuries.

Louis Pasteur (1822–95) and Robert Koch (1843–1910) were twin peaks in the nineteenth-century landscape of microbiology. Their work began an explosion in the discovery of microorganisms as the causative agents of infectious diseases. These discoveries led in turn to new options for the prevention (vaccines, infection control) and treatment (antibiotics) of specific infectious diseases—and moves towards the greater medicalization of public health.[46]

Pasteur's experimental tests of germ theory (first postulated in the sixteenth century) rapidly generated germ facts. Techniques for staining bacteria made them observable under a light microscope. 'Pasteurization' sterilized fermenting liquids by heat-killing microorganisms. Inoculation experiments with killed or attenuated bacteria and viruses produced prototype vaccines against anthrax, chicken cholera, and rabies. Koch's focus was on microbiology to improve public health measures, including sanitation.[47] Based on his work with anthrax, he devised a set of widely used criteria (Koch's postulates) for inferring that a particular microorganism caused a particular disease. The microorganism must be found in diseased but not healthy persons; cultured from a diseased person; cause disease when inoculated into a healthy person; and be recovered from that person. These criteria guided his work to identify the bacteria that caused cholera (as proposed by Filippo Pacini in 1854) and tuberculosis (TB). Experimental microbiology was extended to insect-borne diseases too. Patrick Manson (1844–1922) demonstrated in 1877 that *Culex* mosquitoes are vectors of filarial worms (*Wuchereria*) and Ronald Ross (1857–1932) in 1897 that *Anopheles* mosquitoes transmitted malaria parasites (*Plasmodium*).

The rapid discovery of antibacterial agents gave many more options for treatment: antitoxin or serum therapy for diphtheria (1890), arsenic-derived salvarsan for syphilis (1911), and the true antibiotics (derived from bacteria and fungi) penicillin (1928), sulphonamides (1935), streptomycin (1944), cephalosporins (1945), and tetracycline (1948). But the options for prevention multiplied too, with vaccines for human cholera (1885), typhoid (1896), TB (1921), yellow fever (1936), whooping cough (1939), and Japanese encephalitis (1944).

The causes of the causes

This proliferation of vaccines and antibiotics provided medical reinforcements in the front-line fight against infectious diseases, backed up by large-scale public health measures, and underpinned by improving social and economic conditions. In the first half of the twentieth century, infectious diseases were clearly in decline, but which of these factors was responsible?

The most debated framing of that question was due to a professor of social medicine, Thomas McKeown (1912–88), who observed between the

1950s and 1970s that 'health has advanced significantly only since the late eighteenth century and until recently owed little to medical advances'.[48] McKeown argued that the medical profession had attributed too much of the health benefits to its own work—curative medicine—and commandeered disproportionate resources to do so.[48,49] He pointed instead to the effects of market-based economic growth, the rise in living standards, improved nutrition (the basis of host resistance to infection), and, to a lesser extent, municipal sanitation.[50,51]

Just after World War II, when McKeown began to develop his ideas, recently discovered medical treatments could not possibly account for the decline in infections observed over the preceding decades. The mortality rate from TB in England and Wales had fallen from 320/100,000 population in 1870 to 57/100,000 in 1944 (i.e. by about 80%) when the first TB drug, streptomycin, became available (the BCG vaccine, created in 1921, was not efficacious against infectious pulmonary TB in adults).[52] Deaths from diphtheria, scarlet fever, and pneumonia had also declined before the discovery of antitoxin, sulfa drugs, and penicillin.[53] In McKeown's view, too much credit went to treatment and too little to prevention.

The shortcomings of McKeown's own analyses and conclusions are now well known; he probably overstated the benefits of economic growth and understated the impact of public health measures, especially sanitation.[50] But his question was crucial and stimulated many subsequent investigations, which refined and revised his theory. Samuel Preston (1943–) elevated the role of public health technologies, including water and sanitation, in preventing infections and enhancing life expectancy.[48,54] Robert Fogel (1926–2013) described the positive association between health (measured by height) and nutrition running over two centuries.[55,56] Fogel also saw positive feedbacks between health and human capital: he argued that better nutrition enabled people to grow bigger, stronger, and perhaps smarter, which further boosted income, productivity, and health (Figure 1.1).[57,58]

At the time of McKeown's analysis, preventive measures, whether more (sanitation) or less direct (nutrition), had taken effect over decades. Vaccines and antibiotics had had far less time to make an impact. It is clear now, however, that antibiotics have been responsible for dramatic reductions in mortality (cure), if not the incidence of disease (prevention). For instance, TB deaths per capita declined at only 2%–3%/year in England and Wales between 1870 and 1944. But, thanks to streptomycin, isoniazid, and other TB drugs, the TB death rate dropped far more quickly from the 1940s onwards—by more than 80% within the decade 1946–55 (>15%/year; Figure 1.2).[52]

Other analyses have also revealed that relatively slow gains were made from prevention. In the United States during the 1990s, the preventive measures then in place were extending life expectancy by 18–19 months, less than half as much as the prolongation of life from curative measures, roughly 44–45 months.[59] By these criteria, cure was better than prevention.McKeown had fashioned his argument around the decline in infectious diseases, which were slowly being replaced by chronic, non-communicable diseases in aging populations—the joint epidemiological and demographic transition. Chronic diseases presented the same question about prevention versus treatment, albeit in a new context. Geoffrey Rose's (1926–93) influential *Strategy of Preventive Medicine* (1992)[60–62] drew

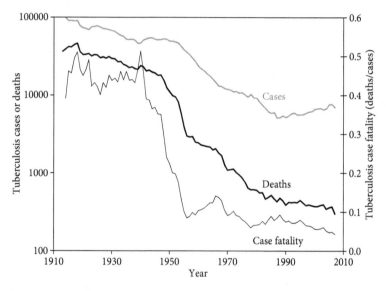

Figure 1.2 Trends in tuberculosis (TB) cases and deaths (left axis) and case fatality (right axis) in England and Wales, 1913–2007. Like other infectious diseases, TB was in decline long before the discovery of antibiotics. From the 1940s onwards, curative drugs greatly accelerated the decline, especially of case fatality (proportion of patients who die), far exceeding the effects of earlier preventive measures. Drug treatment also interrupted transmission and was therefore a means of prevention.

Reproduced with permission from Dye, C. (2015). *The Population Biology of Tuberculosis*. Princeton, USA: Princeton University Press.

attention to the importance of considering risk across whole populations. Taking high blood pressure as a 'risk factor' for stroke, Rose pointed to the potential benefits of changing the behaviour of many people at low risk of illness rather than, or in addition to, targeting a few individuals at high risk. In doing so, his analysis also drew attention to some of the perennial challenges of prevention. Because most diseases are unevenly distributed in populations, population-wide interventions may bring large benefits to an entire population but small benefits to most individuals. For the latter, even a small cost of participation, or a small risk that treatment is harmful, could outweigh the benefits, discouraging compliance.

The investigation of social and economic factors that influence health has a long tradition.[48] Initiatives, such as the World Health Organization (WHO)'s Commission on the Social Determinants of Health (2008), have driven action on 'the causes of the causes'[63] from an explicitly ideological position. In the view of this Commission, health inequalities are unfair and putting them right is a matter of social justice.[64] That ethical position echoes the constitution of WHO where 'the highest attainable standard of health is one of the fundamental rights of every human being'.[65] A weakness of the ideological approach, however, lies in an unwillingness to understand alternative values and viewpoints, when progress actually hinges on such an understanding.[66] To make ideology work, it must be turned into instruments of enticement (carrots: financial and other rewards) or censure (sticks: laws, regulations, social customs), or both.[67] Broadly speaking, the enticements are to promote health, the censures are to prevent illness, but both have leverage (Chapter 6).

There are other reasons why the case for investing in the social, economic, and environmental determinants of health needs to be carefully constructed: although these factors account for as much as 45%–60% of the variation in health in populations around the world (Preface), the benefits of tackling them compared with, say, vaccination or reducing blood pressure, are generally less certain and realized over longer timescales. Despite much promotion, action on the social determinants of health has been less effective than hoped. Successes have been local rather than global, for various reasons: an inward-looking medical focus on health service coverage, commercial conflicts with health, and an equity agenda that does not necessarily appeal to the public or to policymakers.[66]

The questions at the heart of the McKeown debate—prevention versus treatment, market economics versus publicly funded state intervention—remain alive and relevant today. These questions apply just as much to environmental health risks as to those linked to society and the economy.[68]

Environmental becomes existential

As the human population surpassed three billion around 1960, it was becoming clear that none of the earth's life support systems would be free from human influence. The airs, waters, and places of Hippocrates' world were largely fixed sources of risk or benefit to health. Now all natural resources were being shaped by human activity, in all parts of the planet, with big consequences for health and well-being.

Rachel Carson's (1907–64) *Silent Spring* (1962) was a gospel for the new age of concern about mankind's impact on the environment. Carson persuaded a worldwide audience that the indiscriminate use of pesticides was not only poisoning the environment: it was also poisoning people.

Carson contributed to the invention of 'environment' as a political force. *Silent Spring* was a potent influence on a succession of international conferences that made the connection, systematically and systemically, between environment and health. The United Nations Conference on the Human Environment (Stockholm, 1972) proclaimed that 'Man is both creature and moulder of his environment'. The ensuing Stockholm Declaration listed the preventable environmental risks to physical, mental, and social health, specifically 'dangerous levels of pollution, disturbances to the ecological balance of the biosphere, and the depletion of irreplaceable resources'.

The impetus generated in Stockholm was maintained by the 1987 Report of the World Commission on Environment and Development (also known as 'the Brundtland Commission'), which proposed that sustainable development should 'meet the needs of the present without compromising the ability of future generations to meet their own needs'.[69] This definition of sustainability, still used today, laid down a criterion for investing in *Our Common Future*, and for preserving the health and well-being of future generations. As in the Stockholm conference, the Brundtland Commission took a systemic, holistic view of development by framing poverty, inequality, and environmental degradation as interdependent challenges.

The goal of the Earth Summit (Rio de Janeiro, 1992) was to promote international cooperation on the environment after the end of the Cold War. Its main product, the *Rio Declaration on Environment and Development*, embraced the precautionary principle, which had previously been central to the *Montreal Protocol on Substances that Deplete the Ozone Layer* (1987). In the face of future uncertainty, the precautionary principle looks, at first sight, like a strong argument for prevention.[70] Whereas physicians treating individual patients are under oath to 'above all, do no harm',[71] the precautionary principle says, in effect, 'above all, *allow* no harm'. Both principles aim to avoid errors in the face of uncertainty. However, both are ambiguous in practice because decisions, whether they concern the well-being of individuals, populations, or the environment, should balance costs against benefits. For the precautionary principle, to propose safeguards for prevention is not likely to be persuasive unless the benefits (time-discounted and risk-adjusted) outweigh the costs.

Against this historical background, it is widely recognized that the social, economic, environmental, and ethical factors affecting health are interdependent. And yet, in practice, each of these preventable risks to health has been pursued separately, championed, for example, by different intergovernmental organizations: poverty (World Bank), environment (United Nations Environment Programme), food (Food and Agriculture Organization), zoonotic diseases (World Organisation for Animal Health), and health services (WHO).

While specialization gave energy and identity to each technical domain, it neglected the benefits of synergy and connectivity. At the end of the twentieth century, it was time to draw together the separate strands of development to create a comprehensive programme for human health and well-being. 'Ecological public health'[72] might, by cross-linking causes and effects, reinvigorate the agenda for prevention in the twenty-first century— the age of sustainable development.

Prevention for sustainable development

Now, early in the twenty-first century, the United Nations has already set two successive sets of goals based on two different propositions for development: the Millennium Development Goals (MDGs 2000–15) and the Sustainable Development Goals (SDGs 2016–30).[73] The SDGs, more than the MDGs, are a potentially powerful force for prevention.

Three of the eight MDGs were linked to health, focusing on mothers, children, and infectious diseases. The health goals were treated separately from each other and from the other five. They were each to be achieved through top-down, prescriptive, time-limited programmes targeting major causes of illness and death in low- and middle-income countries. Not all goals were met but substantial gains were made: the number of people living in extreme poverty; the malaria, TB, and under-five mortality rates; and the maternal mortality ratio all fell by about one-half or more between 1990 and 2015.[74]

The success of these targeted health programmes was attributed to the provision of medical technologies such as vaccines and drugs. But these successes also relied on functioning health services, run by skilled health workers with health information systems, supply chains, and financing and governance mechanisms. Health gains also depended on social, economic, and environmental factors that lie outside the control of the health sector, such as female education and fertility, family income, and access to safe water and sanitation.[74] This restatement of root causes was integral to the MDG upgrade—the fully comprehensive 2030 Agenda for Sustainable Development.[74] Linked to that Agenda, the 17 SDGs open up new opportunities for development in general and for prevention in particular, tackling the root causes of ill health on all temporal and spatial scales.[75,76]

The transition from MDGs to SDGs requires a cultural change that could take a generation or more. The transition has, in effect, rekindled the McKeown debate. Some experts have argued for maintaining the momentum achieved under the targeted approach. The Copenhagen Consensus Center published in 2015 *The Nobel Laureates' Guide to the Smartest Targets for the World*, still arguing for specific objectives to maximize impact, such as 'lower chronic child malnutrition by 40%', and 'increase immunization, reduce child deaths by 25%'. This chimes with the views of some health professionals who believe that the 'unfinished agenda' of child survival is best served by doing more of what the MDGs prescribed: investing in the immediate benefits of primary health care, rather than in the less certain and slowly realized benefits of, for instance, female education.[77] The argument to 'create fair employment and good work for all'[64] as a basis for better health presents a far greater challenge than, say, 'vaccinate all girls aged 12–18 years against human papilloma virus to protect them from cervical cancer'.[78] In fact, the two approaches should be complementary rather than mutually exclusive, as envisioned by the 2030 Agenda to achieve the SDGs. There is no need, in principle, to choose between prevention and cure, but limited resources might force a choice in practice (Chapter 3).

The principal new goal for health, SDG 3, aims 'to ensure healthy lives and promote well-being for all at all ages'. Universal Health Coverage (UHC), seen as central to achieving SDG 3, means that all individuals and communities receive the health services they need without suffering financial hardship.[79] However, it is under the umbrella of UHC, sitting mainly within the health sector, that 96% of health funding is invested in treatment and only 4% in prevention (Preface, Chapter 3). The advantage of UHC is that it responds to the huge demand for health services: at least half of the world's population still do not have full coverage of essential health services. The disadvantage is that it places less emphasis on tackling the preventable, root causes of ill health, which reside in the other 16 SDGs.

Pay now, live later?

From ancient sanitary systems to contemporary development goals, the circumstances of disease prevention have changed radically over five millennia. The number of people on Earth has increased by a factor of a thousand (from about 7 million to 7 billion); lifespan has more than doubled; the principal causes of death have shifted from infectious diseases in young populations to chronic diseases in aging populations; there is vastly greater understanding of the causes and effects of illness and death, opening up an array of opportunities for intervention; the practice of public health, and the need for collective action, now occur on greatly expanded geographical (from provincial to planetary) and temporal scales (from weeks to centuries).

And yet the underlying principles of prevention—whether applied to personal, social, economic, or environmental health—have remained the same. Throughout history, aspirations to good health have faced the down-to-earth reality that benefits usually come at a cost—hope is free, but expectation has a price tag.

This historical overview, like most others concerning public health, has centred on Europe. But the conditions for staying healthy are the same everywhere: prevention (of any kind of adverse event) should hold most appeal when a reasoning decision maker is asked to pay a small amount while healthy, for an intervention of proven efficacy, against the likely occurrence, in the near future, of an event that is perceived to be serious, such as grave personal illness. Those who pay for prevention want to be assured that the benefits will go to the intended recipients, especially when contributing to collective action for the common good. They should be more willing to pay in advance when avoiding future harm also comes with immediate benefits—such as fresh airs, clean waters, and safe places.

If there is a choice between acting sooner (prevention) or later (treatment and cure), under what conditions will those who have the power to decide favour the former over the latter? By understanding these conditions, is it possible to shift the balance towards staying healthy, or becoming even healthier? Informed by the past, the next step is to lay out a logical framework for investigating prevention—a theory of thinking ahead (Chapter 2).

Summary

The main ideas about preventing illness run through the whole of human history even if, in every age and in every place, they find new interpretation. Spanning 5,000 years, this chapter reveals prevention's common themes, including the following: illnesses have preventable causes (Neolithic filtration and boiling of water); the choice of prevention over cure is conditional on the balance of costs and benefits, where the benefits depend on the risk, timing, and severity of the hazard (shipping insurance, from 4000 BC); prevention is about improving health, not merely avoiding illness (Ancient Greece); prevention is for communal as well as personal health (Roman aqueducts and communal toilets); prevention is at a premium in the absence of a cure (fourteenth-century plague); the costs and benefits of prevention can be calculated and used to make choices about health (Franklin on fire insurance, Chadwick on sanitation); and the immediate, preventable causes of illness (diet, tobacco) depend, in turn, on deeper causes, in societies, economies, and environments (Hippocrates to the SDGs).

References

1. de Roode JC, Lefevre T, Hunter MD. Self-medication in animals. *Science* 2013; *340*: 150–1.
2. Shurkin J. Animals that self-medicate. *Proceedings of the National Academy of Sciences of the United States of America* 2014; *111*: 17339–41.
3. Castella G, Chapuisat M, Christe P. Prophylaxis with resin in wood ants. *Animal Behaviour* 2008; *75*: 1591–6.
4. Brütsch T, Chapusiat M. Wood ants protect their brood with tree resin. *Animal Behaviour* 2014; *93*: 157–61.

5. Zito M, Evans S, Weldon PJ. Owl monkeys (*Aotus* spp.) self-anoint with plants and millipedes. *Folia Primatologica (Basel)* 2003; *74*: 159–61.
6. World Health Organization (WHO) and United Nations Children's Fund. *Progress on Drinking Water, Sanitation and Hygiene: 2017 Update and SDG Baselines.* Geneva: World Health Organization; 2017.
7. Mithen S. *Thirst: Water and Power in the Ancient World.* London: Weidenfeld and Nicholson; 2012.
8. Rosen G. *A History of Public Health.* New York: MD Publications; 1958.
9. Wilson A. Drainage and sanitation. In: Wikander Ö, ed. *Handbook of Ancient Water Technology (Technology and Change in History).* Leiden: EJ Brill; 2000: 151–79.
10. Tankersley KB, Dunning NP, Carr C, Lentz DL, Scarborough VL. Zeolite water purification at Tikal, an ancient Maya city in Guatemala. *Scientific Reports* 2020; *10*: Article number: 18021.
11. Rochberg F. Science and Ancient Mesopotamia. In: Taub AJL, ed. *The Cambridge History of Science.* Cambridge: Cambridge University Press; 2018: 7–28.
12. Kleisiaris CF, Sfakianakis C, Papathanasiou IV. Health care practices in ancient Greece: The Hippocratic ideal. *Journal of Medical Ethics and History of Medicine* 2014; *7*: 6.
13. Tountas Y. The historical origins of the basic concepts of health promotion and education: The role of ancient Greek philosophy and medicine. *Health Promotion International* 2009; *24*: 185–92.
14. Porter D. *Health, Civilisation and the State: A History of Public Health from Ancient to Modern Times.* Abingdon: Routledge; 1999.
15. Hill Curth L. Lessons from the past: Preventive medicine in early modern England. *Medical Humanities* 2003; *29*: 16–20.
16. Brand N. *The Concept of the* Sanus Homo *in the* De Medicina *of Celsus.* Stellenbosch: University of Stellenbosch; 2007.
17. Haueter NV. *A History of Insurance.* Zurich: Swiss Reinsurance Company Ltd; 2017.
18. Buckham D, Wahl J, Rose S. The evolution of insurance. In: *Executive's Guide to Solvency II.* Cary, North Carolina: SAS Institute Inc.; 2010: 1–9.
19. Jacquart D. Anatomy, physiology, and medical theory. In: Lindberg D, Shank M, eds. *The Cambridge History of Science.* Cambridge: Cambridge University Press; 2013: 590–610.
20. Hin S. Mortality. In: *The Demography of Roman Italy: Population Dynamics in an Ancient Conquest Society (201 BCE–14 CE).* Cambridge: Cambridge University Press; 2013: 101–71.
21. Kelishadi R, Hatami H. Avicenna as the forerunner of preventive medicine: On the occasion of 1032nd birth anniversary of Avicenna (22 August 980). *International Journal of Preventive Medicine* 2012; *3*: 517–19.
22. Sairisi NG. *Medieval and Early Renaissance Medicine: An Introduction to Knowledge and Practice.* Chicago: University of Chicago Press; 1990.
23. Barker W. *The Adages of Erasmus.* Toronto: University of Toronto Press; 1500.
24. Cogan T. *The Haven of Health.* London: Roger Ball; 1612.

25. Facts and Details. Nero, Christians, the Great Fire, the rebuilding of Rome and his death. 2019. factsanddetails.com/world/cat56/sub368/entry-6271.html (accessed 7 January 2021).

26. Rogers EM. *Diffusion of Innovations*. 5th edn. New York: Free Press; 2003.

27. Weiss RA, Esparza J. The prevention and eradication of smallpox: A commentary on Sloane (1755) 'An account of inoculation'. *Philosophical Transactions of the Royal Society B* 2015; 370.

28. Grundy I. *Montagu, Lady Mary Wortley*. Oxford: Oxford University Press; 2004.

29. Best M, Katamba A, Neuhauser D. Making the right decision: Benjamin Franklin's son dies of smallpox in 1736. *Quality and Safety in Health Care* 2007; *16*: 478–80.

30. Handman E. Leishmaniasis: Current status of vaccine development. *Clinical Microbiology Reviews* 2001; *14*: 229–43.

31. Porter D. *Health, Civilization and the State: A History of Public Health from Ancient to Modern Times*. London and New York: Routledge; 1999–01.

32. Hamlin C, Sheard S. Revolutions in public health: 1848, and 1998? *BMJ* 1998; *317*: 587–91.

33. Lutz W. Global Sustainable Development priorities 500 y after Luther: *Sola schola et sanitate*. *Proceedings of the National Academy of Sciences of the United States of America* 2017; *114*: 6904–13.

34. Black M, Fawcett B. *The Last Taboo: Opening the Door on the Global Sanitation Crisis*. London: Earthscan; 2008.

35. Dye C. 200 years in the history of longevity. *The Biologist* 2010; *57*: 127–30.

36. Dye C. After 2015: Infectious diseases in a new era of health and development. *Philosophical Transactions of the Royal Society B: Biological Sciences* 2014; *369*: 20130426.

37. Bloy M. Edwin Chadwick (1800–1890). 2002. http://www.victorianweb.org/history/chad1.html (accessed 7 January 2021).

38. van Oosten R. The Dutch Great Stink: The end of the cesspit era in the pre-industrial towns of Leiden and Haarlem. *European Journal of Archaeology* 2016; *19*: 704–27.

39. Acheson RM. Henry Wyldbore Rumsey and the case for state medicine. *Public Health* 1988; *102*: 217–25.

40. Watkins DE. *The English Revolution in Social Medicine, 1889–1911*. London: University of London; 1984.

41. Simon J. *English Sanitary Institutions, Reviewed in their Course of Development, and in some of their Political and Social Relations*. London: Cassell & Company; 1890.

42. Chadwick E. *Report on the Sanitary Conditions of the Labouring Population of Great Britain: A Supplementary Report on the Results of a Special Inquiry into the Practice of Interment in Towns*. London: Poor Law Commissioners; 1843.

43. Joshi P. Edwin Chadwick's self-fashioning: Professionalism, masculinity, and the Victorian poor. *Victorian Literature and Culture* 2004; *32*: 353–70.

44. Tynan N. Nineteenth century London water supply: Processes of innovation and improvement. *The Review of Austrian Economics* 2013; *26*: 73–91.

45. Smith GD. Commentary: Behind the Broad Street pump: Aetiology, epidemiology and prevention of cholera in mid-19th century Britain. *International Journal of Epidemiology* 2002; *31*: 920–32.
46. Worboys M. Public and environmental health. In: Pickstone PBJ, ed. *The Cambridge History of Science*. Cambridge: Cambridge University Press; 2009: 141–64.
47. Ullmann A. Pasteur–Koch: Distinctive ways of thinking about infectious diseases. *Microbe* 2007; *2*: 383–7.
48. Szreter S. The population health approach in historical perspective. *American Journal of Public Health* 2003; *93*: 421–31.
49. McKeown T. *The Role of Medicine: Dream, Mirage, or Nemesis?* London: Nuffield Provincial Hospitals Trust; 1976.
50. Szreter S. Rethinking McKeown: The relationship between public health and social change. *American Journal of Public Health* 2002; *92*: 722–5.
51. Link BG, Phelan JC. McKeown and the idea that social conditions are fundamental causes of disease. *American Journal of Public Health* 2002; *92*: 730–2.
52. Dye C. *The Population Biology of Tuberculosis*. Princeton: Princeton University Press; 2015.
53. Bynum LJ. Riding the waves: Optimism and realism in the treatment of TB. *Lancet* 2012; *380*: 1465–6.
54. Preston SH. *Mortality Patterns in National Populations: With Special Reference to Recorded Causes of Death*. New York: Academic Press; 1976.
55. Fogel RW. *The Escape from Hunger and Premature Death, 1700–2100: Europe, America and the Third World*. Cambridge: Cambridge University Press; 2004.
56. Deaton A. The great escape: A review essay on Fogel's 'The Escape from Hunger and Premature Death, 1700–2100'. *Journal of Economic Literature* 2006; *44*: 106–14.
57. Fogel RW. Health, nutrition, and economic growth. *Economic Development and Cultural Change* 2004; *52*: 643–58.
58. Deaton A. *The Great Escape. Health, Wealth, and the Origins of Inequality*. Princeton and Oxford: Princeton University Press; 2013.
59. Bunker JP, Frazier HS, Mosteller F. Improving health: Measuring effects of medical care. *Milbank Quarterly* 1994; *72*: 225–58.
60. Rose GA. *Rose's Strategy of Preventive Medicine: The Complete Original Text*. Oxford: Oxford University Press; 2008.
61. Charlton BG. A critique of Geoffrey Rose's 'population strategy' for preventive medicine. *Journal of the Royal Society of Medicine* 1995; *88*: 607–10.
62. Rose G. Strategy of prevention: Lessons from cardiovascular disease. *British Medical Journal (Clinical Research Edition)* 1981; *282*: 1847–51.
63. Marmot M. Social determinants of health inequalities. *Lancet* 2005; *365*: 1099–104.
64. Marmot M. *Fair Society, Healthy Lives: The Marmot Review: Strategic Review of Health Inequalities in England Post-2010*. London: Marmot Review Team.
65. World Health Organization. *Constitution of the World Health Organization*. Geneva: WHO; 2006.

66. Rasanathan K. 10 years after the Commission on Social Determinants of Health: Social injustice is still killing on a grand scale. *Lancet* 2018; *392*: 1176–7.

67. de Sadeleer N. *The Principle of Prevention. Environmental Principles: From Political Slogans to Legal Rules.* Oxford: Oxford University Press; 2002.

68. Colgrove J. The McKeown thesis: A historical controversy and its enduring influence. *American Journal of Public Health* 2002; *92*: 725–9.

69. World Commission on Environment and Development. *Our Common Future.* Oxford: United Nations World Commission on Environment and Development (WCED); 1987.

70. Greenhalgh T, Schmid MB, Czypionka T, Bassler D, Gruer L. Face masks for the public during the covid-19 crisis. *BMJ* 2020; *369*: m1435.

71. Smith CM. Origin and uses of *primum non nocere*—above all, do no harm! *Journal of Clinical Pharmacology* 2005; *45*: 371–7.

72. Lang T, Rayner G. Ecological public health: The 21st century's big idea? *BMJ* 2012; *345*: e5466.

73. United Nations. *The Sustainable Development Goals Report.* New York: United Nations; 2018.

74. Dye C. Expanded health systems for sustainable development. *Science* 2018; *359*: 1337–9.

75. International Council for Science (ICSU). *A Guide to SDG Interactions: From Science to Implementation.* Paris: ICSU; 2017.

76. Nilsson M, Griggs D, Visbeck M. Map the interactions between Sustainable Development Goals. *Nature* 2016; *534*: 320–2.

77. Bryce J, Victora CG, Black RE. The unfinished agenda in child survival. *Lancet* 2013; *382*: 1049–59.

78. National Health Service. Who should have the HPV vaccine? 2017. https://www.nhs.uk/conditions/vaccinations/who-should-have-hpv-cervical-cancer-cervarix-gardasil-vaccine (accessed 7 January 2021).

79. World Health Organization. Universal health coverage (UHC). 2019. https://www.who.int/news-room/fact-sheets/detail/universal-health-coverage-(uhc) (accessed 7 January 2021).

2
The problem of prevention

Price is what you pay, value is what you get.

Warren Buffet, after Ben Graham (2009)[1]

Any episode of illness or instance of injury is a failure of prevention. Most people want to lead healthy lives but preventing illness comes at a cost—measured in money, time, effort, information, and willpower, among other kinds of expenditure. In deciding whether to invest in prevention, or take a chance on sickness and cure, a reasoning person will weigh the costs against the benefits. There are standard economic methods for measuring costs and benefits, but choices about health are usually based on the way subjective values are assigned to objective facts.

The 10 greatest achievements of public health in the twentieth century were, according to the US Centers for Disease Control and Prevention: vaccination, motor vehicle safety, safer workplaces, control of infectious diseases, decline in deaths from coronary heart disease and stroke, safer and healthier foods, lower maternal and child mortality, family planning, fluoridation of drinking water, and the recognition of tobacco as a health hazard (cf. sanitation as the greatest achievement since 1840; Chapter 7).[2] Prevention is central to all of them. The questions that motivate this book are: how were these successes achieved, and how can they be extended to other settings?

Rational choice

Any reasoning individual or group of individuals, faced with a risk of illness or death, must decide whether to intervene earlier (prevention) or

The Great Health Dilemma. Christopher Dye, Oxford University Press. © Oxford University Press 2021. DOI: 10.1093/oso/9780198853824.003.0002

later (cure), balancing the pros and cons of each option. If prevention is not thought to be better than cure, there should be a discernible reason why.

To investigate the basis of choice is an explicitly 'positive' approach to the economics of decision making.[3] Positive means beginning with an impartial, descriptive study of how and why things are as we see them—leading to a testable hypothesis—rather than with prescriptive or 'normative' judgements of how they should be seen.[4] The literature in public health economics is dominated by prescription and underserved by description. One reason for this is that governments are primary customers for economic evaluation, and commonly seek advice on how best to allocate limited resources to health care. For instance, a public health service often needs to answer a single question on behalf of a single group of people, based on standard methods of assessing costs and benefits.[5,6] The kind of question asked is: which of two antibiotics, doxycycline or azithromycin, is more cost-effective in preventing sexually transmitted infections between partners?[7] Or, with what risk of heart disease should patients become eligible to receive drugs that lower blood pressure?[8] Cost-effectiveness analysis, and related forms of economic evaluation, give useful results under these particular circumstances—when they are the predetermined method of decision making (Box 2.1).

But decisions are not always, or even usually, made in ways that would be predicted by standard appraisals in health economics. Consider, for example, the decisions made by governments in low- and middle-income countries to adopt vaccines that prevent pneumococcal and rotavirus infections, the causes of pneumonia and diarrhoea. Economic evaluations find that these vaccines are cost-effective in countries that still have high levels of child mortality.[9] But there are other criteria for choosing vaccines. One study of seven low-income countries found that the choice of when and which vaccines to adopt was guided partly by cost-effectiveness, but also by related and unanticipated derivatives of it: short-term costs; funding available from the Global Alliance on Vaccines and Immunization (GAVI); estimates of the burden of disease to be overcome; and local political priorities.[10-12] The decision to adopt a vaccine was not based on the feasibility of adding it to immunization schedules, or on financial sustainability. And it did not depend, apparently, on whether preventing pneumonia and diarrhoeal disease was thought to be better than treating these conditions in children. In short, the governments of these seven countries were not always framing their choices in the way presumed by standard economic evaluation. Nor were they explicitly asking whether prevention was better

Box 2.1 Accounting for health

The International Classification of Diseases is a system of medical codes—55,000 codes in the 11th revision (ICD-11)—created by the World Health Organization (WHO) to classify diagnoses, diseases, signs and symptoms, and the social circumstances of illness and death. Standard definitions in ICD-11 are the basis for measuring health and well-being in populations, in broadly three ways:

1. Single measures of health. The primary statistics of epidemiological studies include the number of new cases of illness per unit time (incidence), the number of cases of illness at any given time (prevalence), and the number of deaths per unit time (mortality). To help explain the distribution of health and disease in populations, incidence, prevalence, and mortality are categorized by person (age, sex, ethnicity, etc.), place (geographical location) and time (days, months, years), and with reference to the denominator population size. Secondary measures of health and disease in populations can be derived from primary records of cases and deaths, such as life expectancy from birth or deaths by age.

2. Compound measures of health. The magnitude of a health problem in a population, and the choice of a solution, are judged absolutely and comparatively. To aid comparisons between diseases with different effects on health, methods have been devised to put illness and death in the same currency. One standard metric, the quality-adjusted life year (QALY), is equivalent to one year of life in perfect health. QALYs are intended to measure health gains—for example, when tracking patients in clinical trials who, following treatment, live for a number of years with each year weighted by a quality-of-life score on a scale of 0–1. Quality of life is typically measured in terms of a patient's ability to carry out daily activities with freedom from pain and mental disturbance, but QALYs emphasize health rather than quality of life more broadly. In contrast, the disability-adjusted life year (DALY) measures health losses and is favoured in studies of disease burden. One DALY is a year of healthy life lost due to illness or injury, calculated as years lost to illness × disability weight + years lost by death. QALYs and DALYs are standardized measures of utility but exclude many factors that influence subjective values of health and well-being, as described in the main text. There are numerous reasons to be careful when computing and comparing health outcomes with QALYs and DALYs. For instance, quantitative values

assigned to the quality of life and disability are debatable. Also questionable is the proposition that disability can be equated with death (e.g. that 5×0.2 (disability weight) years of blindness = 1 year of life lost = 1 DALY). Death is a qualitatively different condition from disability, which is a reason for keeping the two measures separate.

Among the most frequently used tools in economic evaluation, cost-effectiveness analysis (CEA) compares the costs of an intervention against the effects measured with simple (deaths averted) or compound (QALYs gained, etc.) measures of health. In the UK, the National Institute for Health and Care Excellence (NICE) considers a threshold of less than £20,000–£30,000 per QALY gained to be cost-effective for the National Health Service.[1] A threshold US$50,000–US$150,000 per QALY has been used in the United States. WHO recommends that the cost per DALY should be less than the national per capita gross domestic product. Such benchmarks are convenient, and absolute values of costs (maximum affordable cost) and benefits (minimum desirable effect) are important, but CEA is essentially comparative.

3. Monetary value of health. Appealing to economists, but contentious among health specialists, are methods that put the costs and benefits of prevention or treatment in the same currency—money. A single currency is useful for trading in a diversity of goods, as when considering the effects of prevention on health in the broadest sense (WHO's 'state of complete physical, mental and social well-being') and the effects beyond health (e.g. other Sustainable Development Goals). The dominant method is to calculate the Value of a Statistical Life (VSL) i.e. the amount of money that a person or society is willing to pay to save one anonymous human life. Four main methods are used to compute VSL based on human capital (lost earnings), contingent valuation (willingness to pay to lower the risk of death, or compensation required to accept a higher risk of death), the labour market (wage differentials for jobs that carry different risks of injury or death), and consumer preference (willingness to pay for safety features on consumer products, where cost can be linked to risk of injury or death, e.g. car airbags). The last two are based on de facto 'revealed preferences'. Like QALYs and DALYs, estimates of VSL (e.g. range $7–$12 million for the US labour market) need careful application. For example, an estimate of the benefit/cost ratio > 1 is not, on its own, justification for choosing an intervention. Furthermore, when the monetary benefit and cost are calculated in different ways (e.g. VSL benefit versus cash cost), it is potentially misleading to say that a benefit/cost ratio > 1 is cost-saving.[2]

The ratio of benefit to cost, or the difference ([benefit-cost]/cost, i.e. the return on investment), should be compared with ratios and differences for competing investments, calculated using the same methods.

These standard methods of measurement are generally used comparatively (e.g. to set priorities for intervention), as when comparing methods of prevention and cure. A general rule for choosing among them is to select the most direct measurement of health (such as case incidence), compromising only when it is necessary to make comparisons in the same units (often money).

Economic evaluation, mainly cost-effectiveness analysis, is used to guide government decision makers who are making a single choice about a single problem on behalf of a single population.[3] Economic evaluation is much less useful in showing how, beyond narrowly defined constraints, choices are really made about health, and it is not intended to do so. In general, the challenge for economic evaluation is to put the right value on health—that is, the value that individuals, governments, businesses, and others actually use to make a choice. Because the values are often subjective interpretations of the facts, a code of ethics is needed to define what is right or wrong, from the perspective of a community of people who are making collective decisions.

Source: Data from Social Value UK (2016). *Valuation of a Life*; Drummond MF, Sculpher MJ, Torrance GW et al. (2005). *Methods for the Economic Evaluation of Health Care Programmes.* 3rd edition. Oxford University Press.

Notes:

1. Paulden M. Recent amendments to NICE's value-based assessment of health technologies: Implicitly inequitable? *Expert Review of Pharmacoeconomics and Outcomes Research* 2017; *17*: 239–42.

2. Masters R, Anwar E, Collins B, Cookson R, Capewell S. Return on investment of public health interventions: A systematic review. *Journal of Epidemiology Community Health* 2017; *71*: 827–34.

3. Morgan MG, Kandlikar M, Risbey J, Dowlatabadi H. Why conventional tools for policy analysis are often inadequate for problems of global change. *Climatic Change* 1999; *41*: 271–81.

than cure. This work, following a small number of other studies, highlighted the rarity of investigations into the process of decision making in public health.[13–15]

In 1997, the United Kingdom government was under pressure to relax the pet quarantine law, which required dogs and cats entering the country to be isolated for six months. The purpose of the quarantine law was to prevent the reintroduction of rabies into the UK. Abandoning quarantine would increase the risk, but this could be offset by vaccination. The risk of rabies entering the UK was estimated to lie between 1 in 50 million immigrant pets under the existing quarantine policy, and a maximum of 1 in 10 million with no entry restrictions. However, the politically defined criterion for a new policy framed risk in a different and unexpected way. The new policy should guarantee that the UK would remain rabies-free for at least 20 years. No policy can guarantee a statistical risk of zero; the agreed solution was a vaccination regime that might allow one case in an estimated 28–34 years. This was the basis of the pet travel scheme (PETS) that came into force in year 2000.[16]

These choices about vaccines and vaccination policies were considered rational for those governments at that time. Without understanding the basis of choice, it is difficult to influence it, or even to discuss whether governments are asking the right question in the first place. The lesson for investigators is that a study of how choices are actually made (costs, criteria, constraints, preferences) should be carried out routinely, preceding prescriptive analyses of how they should be made.

'Irrational' choice

When choices about prevention or cure do not conform with expectations, they are often labelled 'irrational'. In view of the factors affecting vaccine adoption (as described in the previous section), a better approach is to investigate the reasons for what appear to be illogical 'false economies'.

One example is the routine use of medical and dental checks, means of (primary) prevention that aim to identify and eliminate risks before they cause disease. The problem with routine health checks is that they are typically offered to people who are mostly at low risk of illness; they tend to be used by those who need them least, and they generally give a poor return on investment.[17] Despite the economic arguments against 'healthy condition monitoring' (Box 2.2), HCM accounted for nearly half of all spending on prevention in Organisation for Economic Co-operation and Development (OECD) countries in 2015.[18–20] In contrast, immunization and screening for specific diseases, which are consistently cost-effective and sometimes cost-saving, attracted less than one fifth of expenditure on prevention.

Box 2.2 International System of Health Accounts (SHA)

By definition, 'prevention is any measure that aims to avoid or reduce the number or the severity of injuries and diseases, their sequelae and complications'.[1,2] In SHA, that definition includes primary prevention (avoiding disease and mitigating risk factors) and secondary prevention (early detection and treatment of disease) but not tertiary prevention (mitigating the effects of established disease or injury), although the principles of prevention described in the main text apply to all three categories.

The main areas of prevention and public health services covered by SHA are: information, education, and counselling; immunization (vaccination); early disease detection (secondary prevention); healthy condition monitoring (e.g. pregnancy, children, dental); epidemiological surveillance, and risk and disease control; and preparing for disasters and emergencies. These cover, partly or wholly, widely recognized Essential Public Health Operations.[3]

In the context of prevention, SHA is limited because it includes only spending for which improving health is the primary purpose.[1] SHA covers, for instance, the cost of developing tobacco legislation by a Ministry of Health (mainly staff costs under 'governance') but not the costs to government of enforcing legislation on tobacco companies, or of managing tobacco industry lobbying. Neither does SHA offset expenditure with revenue from taxes on tobacco sales.[4]

In general, and in terms of the 17 Sustainable Development Goals (SDGs), SHA ignores the benefits to and from health (SDG 3) of the other 16 SDGs (Health in All Policies, HiAP), which set targets for agriculture, education, energy, environment, housing, transport, water and sanitation, and other sectors. SHA does attempt to collect information on 'health promotion with a multi-sectoral approach'[1] but, even within the limited scope of this category, data are reported by few countries. The practical implementation of HiAP would benefit from a systematic financial accounting system for health in the SDGs, but that does not yet exist.[5]

Source: Data from Duran, A., Kutzin, J. Financing of public health services and programmes: time to look into the black box. In: Kutzin J, Cashin C, Jakab M, eds. *Implementing Health Financing Reform.* Copenhagen: World Health Organization; 2010: 247–68; Schmidt H, Gostin LO, Emanuel EJ (2015) Public health, universal health coverage, and Sustainable Development Goals: Can they coexist? *Lancet, 386*: 928–30.

Notes:

1. Organization for Economic Cooperation and Development (OECD), Eurostat, and World Health Organization. *A System of Health Accounts 2011: Revised Edition.* Paris: OECD; 2017.

2. Henderson J. *Expenditure on Prevention Activities under SHA 2011: Supplementary Guidance*. Paris: OECD; 2013.

3. World Health Organization Regional Office for Europe. *The Case for Investing in Public Health*. Copenhagen: World Health Organization Regional Office for Europe; 2014.

4. McDaid D, Sassi F, Merkur S. (eds). *Promoting Health, Preventing Disease: The Economic Case*. Berkshire, UK: McGraw Hill; 2015.

5. Duran A, Kutzin J. Financing of public health services and programmes: Time to look into the black box. In: Kutzin J, Cashin C, Jakab M, eds. *Implementing Health Financing Reform*. Copenhagen: World Health Organization; 2010: 247–68.

The apparently unjustified use of HCM could be explained in a number of ways: routine checks might, for example, offer reassurance about health, which patients are willing to pay for through health insurance. Whatever the reason, the first step is to suppose that there is a discoverable explanation for why HCM still commands such a large fraction of OECD budgets. The explanation might never be found if HCM is rejected on the basis of a narrow set of predetermined normative criteria.

There are plenty of reasons why decisions about health may, at first sight, seem irrational. Deeper investigations of unexpected choices, in a wide variety of contexts, have led to fundamental discoveries about how cultural (ethical, moral, spiritual), psychological (emotional, cognitive, computational, neurological), and social factors (contextual, ethnic) influence decisions, including the way in which different individuals, and different groups of individuals, weigh up costs and benefits to make choices. Some of this work lies in the domains of behavioural economics and finance (humans)[21–25] and behavioural ecology (animals).[26]

Behavioural economics has become a rich source of theories about how to explain apparent misbehaviours, and of ideas about how to change them for the better. The UK government's Behavioural Insights Team aims to make progress through 'radical incrementalism'.[27] The so-called 'Nudge Unit' has, for example, used social norms to encourage the payment of taxes: advertising that most people pay their taxes on time persuades others to do so too. They have improved adherence to tuberculosis (TB) treatment by allowing patients to submit video evidence that they have taken their medication, instead of having to visit a clinic. But these successes do not guarantee others: the proposal that a behavioural nudge can remedy misbehaviour is a testable idea, not an established truth.[21,28]

One category of unexpected choices, among many, is the disproportionate influence of single, major events on decision making. During the early 1950s in London, heavily polluted air was the norm. But it took 'the UK's greatest peacetime disaster',[29] a particularly lethal smog in December

1952, to precipitate the Clean Air Act of 1956, which restricted the use of toxic heating fuels and established smoke-free zones in heavily populated areas.[30] Likewise, cigarette smoking was finally banned on all London Underground trains and stations after the King's Cross fire of 1987.[31] Given the well-known effects of smoking on health, there was mounting pressure for a ban, but the final decision was triggered by fire safety, rather than by the argument that smoking damages health.

Because the value of an outcome is often not an absolute number but a relative one, change from a point of reference is critical.[4] In the United States, after yet another mass shooting (four or more people injured or killed) on 31 May 2019, Senator Elizabeth Warren pointed out that everyday gun violence, which contributes far more deaths annually than mass shooting, is under-reported because it is considered to be normal.[32] On that occasion, thirteen people were shot dead at a government building in Virginia Beach. Putting that mass shooting in context, more than 15,000 people were killed by gun violence in the United States in 2019 and over 19,000 in 2020 (excluding suicides).[33] Clearly, perceptions of what is normal and abnormal, as well as the facts, must inform the 'public health approach' to violent crime. That approach aims to prevent, rather than react to, deaths from guns, knives, and other weapons by asking standard population-based, epidemiological questions about perpetrators and their victims: who, where, when, and why?[34,35]

Strong reactions to rare events with major consequences are the norm rather than the exception.[36] To recognize that fact has the potential to turn public overreactions into more measured political responses that would, for instance, minimize the total number of gun deaths in the US, not just the number of mass shootings.

The characteristics of prevention

Harvey Fineberg identified many of the reasons why prevention is characteristically 'celebrated in principle, resisted in practice'.[37] On his list (with my choice of examples) are the following:

- Population statistics have little emotional impact compared with personal stories: the school groundsman who developed cancer after, though not necessarily because of, long-term exposure to glyphosate weedkiller, a hazard that is 'probably carcinogenic to humans'. [38,39]

- Lasting behaviour changes are needed, which are often difficult to achieve: take regular exercise, choose a healthy diet.[40]
- Commercial interests are detrimental to health: the promotion and sale of alcohol, tobacco, and sugar-sweetened drinks.[41,42]
- Advice runs contrary to personal, religious, or cultural beliefs: after a death from Ebola virus disease, ceremonial contact with the body risks exposure to infection.[43]

But all these reasons could apply to curative treatment too. They offer plausible grounds for not choosing prevention in specific instances. And yet, if prevention is systematically disfavoured, as experience suggests, it must have distinctive features.

Ten of these are listed in Table 2.1, but we can further explore the characteristics of prevention through an example that has been central to the history of public health—the slow and intermittent progress in achieving safe sanitation worldwide (Chapters 1 and 7).

In the professional world of faecal management, the core of Figure 2.1 (in black) is called the 'F-diagram'.[44,45] It maps out faecal–oral routes of infection—the pathways along which pathogens in animal and human faeces, including bacteria, viruses, and parasites, reach the mouths and guts of their human victims—through fluids, fingers, flies, fomites, fields, and floors.

The cardinal virtue of prevention, as compared with treatment, is the intent to avert entire episodes of illness, or at least episodes of serious illness. Interventions earlier in the causal chain (upstream, to the left of Figure 2.1) do this by blocking or removing environmental contamination through animal husbandry, fly control, water purification, sanitation, and drug treatment of infected humans and animals. Upstream interventions have costs and benefits beyond health: toilets can be designed to satisfy preferences, not only for cleanliness and hygiene but also for convenience, dignity, privacy, and safety (in grey). A domestic sanitation system is a household asset, which not only disposes of excreta but can also recycle faecal waste in biofuels and fertilizers, and add value to a property. Water and sanitation infrastructure is costly and delivers health and financial returns slowly, over months and years, so the costs should be set against all the possible benefits.[46]

Interventions further downstream (to the right of Figure 2.1) have more specific but more certain and more immediate benefits for health. Better nutrition through breast feeding, zinc supplements, and nutrient-rich food

Table 2.1 Ten challenges to prevention

Factor[1]	Challenge	Explanation	Example
Hazard (*H*)	Unvalued	Interventions earlier in a causal chain (upstream) have a greater number of effects than later (downstream curative treatment); greater organization is needed to secure all the benefits of acting earlier.	There is insufficient information on the magnitude of interlinked causes and effects to capture the full benefits of prevention e.g. across the Sustainable Development Goals.[2,3]
	Invisible	Successful prevention is less visible than cure (absence of illness); health is not valued until it is lost; some failures of prevention have less impact than others.	Failing to provide clean water is more critical than failing to install a sewage system.[4]
	Unattributable	When ill health has multiple possible causes and prevention fails, it may not be possible to identify who or what was responsible.	Economic austerity is associated with increased mortality, but the evidence for a causal link is not definitive, either for populations or individuals.[5,6]
Risk (*p*)	Unlikely	A proportion of people at risk who will not become ill (identity unknown) are subject to a prophylactic intervention with small benefit (peace of mind) and some cost (including possible harm).	In the wake of COVID-19, the risk of another pandemic might still be considered low, compromising investment in preparedness.[7]
	Uncertain	Uncertainty, including distrust, fosters public unwillingness to follow health recommendations.	Distrust fosters vaccine hesitancy or refusal.[8,9]
Time (*d*)	Untimely	Delayed threats are valued less (time discounted) than imminent ones; rewards obtained with a delay are valued less than those gained immediately; prevention gives way to treatment during emergencies.	In a cholera outbreak, the priority is to detect and treat cases early and monitor water sources, rather than to invest in water and sanitation;[10] delayed rewards are discounted, such as mitigating the effects of climate change[11] or educating girls to improve the health of their future children.[12,13]

Continued

Table 2.1 *Continued*

Factor[1]	Challenge	Explanation	Example
Cost (C)	Ineffective	Intervention efficacy diminishes with more links in a causal chain; per effect, upstream interventions are generally less efficacious than downstream interventions, but have a wider range of effects.	Vaccination is more efficacious than personal hygiene or sanitation in preventing rotavirus infection, but sanitation and hygiene have a wider range of benefits.[14]
Choice	Uncompetitive	Prevention is supplementary to cure in health care services and subsidiary to goals in other sectors.	When health budgets are squeezed, curative medical services are protected before prevention and public health.[15]
	Unfair	Criteria for prevention are more stringent than for cure.	Decision-makers sometimes require prevention to be cost-saving, not merely cost-effective.[16,17–21]
	Unfavourable	Cheap and efficacious cures are a possible disincentive for prevention.	Oral rehydration therapy might diminish the value of sanitation to prevent diarrhoeal diseases.[22,23]

Notes:

1. Factors that can discourage prevention, diminishing the magnitude of a threat through their effects on hazard, risk, time, cost, and on the options that constrain choice. These factors are characteristic of prevention; many more could be listed that apply both to curative treatment as well as prevention, adding to those given in the main text.

2. British Medical Association. *Exploring the Cost Effectiveness of Early Intervention and Prevention*. London: British Medical Association; 2017.

3. The Academy of Medical Sciences. *Improving the Health of the Public by 2040*. London: The Academy of Medical Sciences; 2016.

4. Department for International Development (DFID) Sanitation Reference Group. Sanitation Policy Background Paper. *Water Is Life, Sanitation Is Dignity*. London: DFID; 2007.

5. McDermid V. Is austerity linked to 120,000 unnecessary deaths? 2018. https://fullfact.org/health/austerity-120000-unnecessary-deaths (accessed 16 January 2021).

6. Quilter-Pinner H, Hochlaf D. *Austerity: There is an alternative and the UK can afford to deliver it*. London: Institute for Public Policy Research; 2019.

7. World Health Organization. Ten threats to global health in 2019. 2019. https://www.who.int/news-room/feature-stories/ten-threats-to-global-health-in-2019 (accessed 16 January 2021).

8. Hoffman BL, Felter EM, Chu KH, et al. It's not all about autism: The emerging landscape of anti-vaccination sentiment on Facebook. *Vaccine* 2019; *37*: 2216–23.

9. Goldenberg MJ. Antivaccination movement exploits public's distrust in scientific authority. *BMJ* 2019; *367*: l6960.

Table 2.1 *Continued*

10. Global Task Force on Cholera Control (GTFCC). *Ending Cholera: A Global Roadmap to 2030*. Geneva: World Health Organization; 2018.

11. Nordhaus W. Economics. Critical assumptions in the Stern Review on climate change. *Science* 2007; *317*: 201–2.

12. Bryce J, Victora CG, Black RE. The unfinished agenda in child survival. *Lancet* 2013; *382*: 1049–59.

13. Kuruvilla S, Schweitzer J, Bishai D, et al. Success factors for reducing maternal and child mortality. *Bulletin of the World Health Organization* 2014; *92*: 533–44.

14. Crawford SE, Ramani S, Tate JE, et al. Rotavirus infection. *Nature Reviews Disease Primers* 2017; *3*: 17083.

15. Gmeinder M, Morgan D, Mueller M. *How much Do OECD Countries Spend on Prevention?* Paris: Organisation for Economic Co-operation and Development; 2017.

16. Fineberg HV. The paradox of disease prevention: Celebrated in principle, resisted in practice. *Journal of the American Medical Association* 2013; *310*: 85–90.

17. Hale J, Phillips CJ, Jewell T. Making the economic case for prevention—A view from Wales. *BMC Public Health* 2012; *12*: 460.

18. Buck D. *Talking about the 'Return on Investment of Public Health': Why it's Important to Get it Right*. London: The King's Fund; 2018.

19. Rappange DR, Brouwer WB, Rutten FF, van Baal PH. Lifestyle intervention: From cost savings to value for money. *Journal of Public Health (Oxford Academic)* 2010; *32*: 440–7.

20. Suhrcke M, Urban D, Moesgaard Iburg K, Schwappach D, Boluarte T, McKee M. *The Economic Benefits of Health and Prevention in a High-Income Country: The Example of Germany*. Berlin: Wissenschaftszentrum Berlin für Sozialforschung (WZB); 2007.

21. McGinnis JM, Williams-Russo P, Knickman JR. The case for more active policy attention to health promotion. *Health Affairs (Millwood)* 2002; *21*: 78–93.

22. Nalin DR, Cash RA. 50 years of oral rehydration therapy: The solution is still simple. Lancet 2018; 392: 536–8.

23. World Health Organization. *The WHO Model List of Essential Medicines*, 21st List. Geneva: World Health Organization, 2019.

protects against diarrhoeal diseases and provides long-term health benefits for children and their mothers.[47,48] Immunization prevents infection with pathogens that cause diarrhoea—rotavirus, *Salmonella enterica* 'Typhi' (typhoid), *Vibrio* (cholera), *Shigella* (dysentery), and enterotoxigenic *Escherichia coli* (ETEC)—and helps to break the transmission cycle of these pathogens, but it gives no protection against other causes of diarrhoea.[49–52]

When all these interventions fail to prevent illness (to the far right of Figure 2.1), then curative treatments are needed, such as oral rehydration therapy (ORT). ORT is a cheap, reliable, and rapidly effective remedy for diarrhoea caused by a variety of pathogens, but it does little to interrupt onward transmission.[51,53]

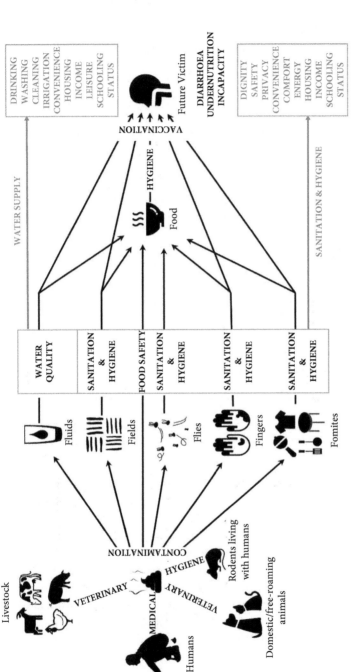

Figure 2.1 The F-diagram (black) of sources of intestinal infections acquired orally from human and animal faeces, and methods of blocking these sources of infection, expanded to include benefits other than health from safe water and sanitation (grey).

Adapted under a Creative Commons Attribution 4.0 International (CC BY 4.0) from Penakalapati, G., Swarthout, J., Delahoy, M.J., *et al.* (2017). Exposure to animal faeces and human health: a systematic review and proposed research priorities. *Environmental Science and Technology.* 51: 11537–52. Adapted under a Creative Commons Attribution 3.0 IGO (CC BY 3.0 IGO) from Hutton, G., Chase, C. Water supply, sanitation, and hygiene. In: Mock, C.N., Nugent, R., Kobusingye, O., Smith, K.R., (eds.)(2017). *Injury Prevention and Environmental Health*: 171–98. Washington DC, USA: World Bank.

This range of options makes clear the trade-offs up and down the causal chain of illness: upstream interventions have a wider range of effects (on costs and benefits), but with less certain outcomes (positive or negative), and act relatively slowly. Downstream interventions have more specific but more certain and more immediate outcomes. In view of these trade-offs, costs and benefits should be judged with respect to particular interventions, rather than in terms of specific risks to health ('risk factors') or health conditions ('hazards'). Adding up all the costs and benefits will determine where best to intervene in the causal chain.

The F-diagram exposes another factor that influences the point of intervention: chance or contingency (Figure 2.1). It is a lucky coincidence, for instance, that rotavirus is a naturally immunizing infection, a factor that enables vaccine development. Or that *S*. Typhi, the agent of typhoid, has restricted routes of transmission that make this pathogen vulnerable to even modest improvements in sanitation. The reservoir for *S*. Typhi is exclusively human, the infectious dose is high compared with other pathogens that cause diarrhoea, and the sources are predominantly water and contaminated food, with little person-to-person transmission.

Finally, when there are options for both prevention and treatment, they are not usually simple alternatives. For instance, ORT should always be available as a treatment until the incidence of diarrhoeal disease is reduced by preventive methods. For diarrhoeal diseases, and for illnesses more generally, prevention will usually be supplementary to cure, rather than an immediate replacement for it. So extra resources have to be found for prevention in health services, until the funding for clinical care is no longer needed (Chapter 3).

These specific aspects of health in relation to sanitation lead to a simple conceptual model of prevention, which can be tested and adapted to a wider variety of settings.

Costs and benefits of prevention: Principles

Value of prevention

The testable idea is this: prevention is more likely to be favoured when a low-cost, high-efficacy intervention can remove a serious hazard to health, definitely and quickly. The expected value of a future threat, $E(V)$, from a given hazard (to health or to any other asset) is usually defined as the product:

$$E(V) = p \times H \qquad (1)$$

H is the magnitude of the hazard. For an individual person, this could be the severity of illness or the probability of death. For a population, it is the severity multiplied by the number of people affected—the population burden of disease. Probability p (range 0–1) is the chance or risk that the hazard will occur. If $p = 0$ there is no risk and the hazard is not a threat. As p increases in size, the threat becomes more likely; it is certain when $p = 1$. In some formulations of the expected threat, p or H allow for the vulnerability of certain populations to particular hazards, but vulnerability is not made explicit here.

Time preference

The future is generally worth less than the present so the value of a threat should be (time) discounted in formula (1).

From an economic perspective, money received in the future, rather than the present, is devalued by the interest that would have been earned on an investment or purchase made now. Health, too, is usually worth more today than in the future. However, the magnitude and form of the time preference varies for different people in different settings facing different health threats, so time preferences and discount rates should be investigated, not simply assumed.[55,56]

Extending formula (1), the expected value today of a threat that might occur at some time in the future becomes:

$$E(V) = p \times d \times H \qquad (2)$$

where d is the discount factor (range 0–1), which is smaller for a threat that is expected in the more distant future. More precisely, the present value of a future threat, $E(V)$, is the sum of the product $p \times d \times H$ over all future times at which the threat could occur.

The goal of prevention is to reduce the threat, $E(V)$, as much as possible and at least cost. The motivation for action will be greatest (large $E(V)$) when facing a large, preventable hazard (big H) that is very likely to happen (p → 1), and soon (d → 1). The most desirable intervention is one that reduces the risk that the hazard will occur and does so quickly. Attached to empirical measurements of risk are estimates of precision or (un)certainty. Uncertainty about the risk, and therefore the value of removing it, generally diminishes the threat and deters prevention.

Formula (2) also applies to medical treatment, so different options for prevention and cure can be compared, subject to constraints on choice. The advantage of primary prevention is that all of the hazard (H) would be averted. The disadvantage is that the hazard is yet to happen, so $p \leq 1$ and $d \leq 1$ For treatment, by comparison, the threat has already occurred: $E(V)$ is bigger because $p = d = 1$, but smaller because treatment removes only a fraction of the hazard, H. So prevention may not be better than cure, but the principles identify the circumstances under which it could be.

Cost of prevention

Value for money comes from minimizing the cost C (per efficacious application) in relation to the expected value of the threat removed, $E(V)$, by prevention or treatment. A consideration of cost puts the focus on the intervention, as previously suggested in the context of sanitation, with at least three implications. First, the benefits should count all the hazard(s) prevented, which may include several different aspects of health and well-being. Second, the costs of prevention and cure will often be different because the methods of prevention (e.g. vaccines) and cure (e.g. drugs), and their efficacies, are also different. Third, the costs and benefits to health providers and consumers also usually differ, so cooperation is needed to resolve conflicts of interest. For instance, health is valued differently by the consumers and manufacturers of tobacco, alcohol, sugary drinks, and salty snacks (Chapter 6).[57] Public health generally succeeds through collective action, although interactions among people with different interests are not made explicit in the simple conceptual model described by formulae (1) and (2) above.

Utility and choice

Each of the elements of $E(V)$, plus the cost (C), can be measured object-ively. The magnitude of a health hazard, H, is usually measured in terms of health (e.g. case fatality), or a compound measure of health (such as quality-adjusted life years [QALYs]), or in terms of money (Box 2.1). Any of these standard measures are satisfactory when there is agreement on the interpretation of value—for instance, when a public health service decides to allocate resources based on the numbers of cases or deaths averted in re-lation to cost.[58]

But that is a special case. More generally, choice is determined by the subjective evaluation (utility) of objective facts. In what might have been the founding statement of utility theory (long predating Warren Buffet's epigram above; Chapter 1), Gabriel Cramer proposed in 1728 that 'math-ematicians estimate money in proportion to its quantity, and men of good sense in proportion to the usage that they may make of it'. In short, choice depends on value as well as price. That idea was captured in tests of Daniel Bernouilli's 1738 'expected utility hypothesis' (rightly, a testable hypoth-esis),[59] and underpins the notion of utility used here too (cf. standardized measures of utility in health, described in Box 2.1).

The perceived value of a health threat, and the choices that are made in the face of that threat, depend on who is doing the valuation—a public or private health provider, or someone who uses their services. And they may all interpret the same statistics in different ways.

Behavioural research has amassed a wealth of information about the way costs, risks, and hazards are perceived.[60,61] The prevention of illness that re-sults in a loss of earnings is more important to those on lower incomes. The costs and benefits of immunization are irrelevant if vaccines are refused on religious grounds. A hazard is not a threat if the chance of illness is thought, through ignorance or misinformation, to be zero. In some circumstances, where knowledge of a health hazard is qualitatively understood, the chance of illness is systematically overestimated, as for the uptake of influenza vac-cination, screening for breast cancer, and aspirin to prevent heart disease, revealed by one study in the Netherlands.[62]

For a given, objective measure of disease severity, such as case fatality, health hazards seem less threatening when they are familiar rather than novel; cause chronic rather than acute illness; are benign rather dreaded (haemorrhagic Ebola, sharks, snakes); affect adults rather than children;

natural rather than man-made; and endemic (steady) rather than epidemic (changing). Change is threatening: a sudden increase in the number of deaths from cholera is taken more seriously than the same number of deaths from other causes of diarrhoea, which change little from year to year.

Risks tend to be downgraded when they are voluntary rather than imposed, predictable rather than unpredictable, pleasurable rather than painful (alcohol, tobacco, sex), controllable rather than uncontrollable (aeroplane accidents), and when they come from a trusted rather than an untrusted source (vaccination). The death of a named patient today caused by a failure of treatment (error of commission) is perceived to be more critical than an anonymous future death caused by a failure of prevention (error of omission).

A hazard is perceived to be more of a threat when close and personal. Most compelling (and honest) are stories about individual people that reflect general truths rather than exceptional (usually bad) experiences. Between 23 June and 10 July 2018, 12 boys and their football coach were trapped in a flooded cave in Thailand, attracting continuous attention from the world's media. It is clear why the incident held a global audience spellbound: they were children, each with character and identity, the rescue was full of daring and suspense, and the Thai authorities were in the spotlight. All 13 were safely rescued. During the same period, 214 anonymous African migrants attempting to cross the Mediterranean drowned in two separate incidents off the Libyan coast. That drew far less attention: such incidents had become routine, and migrant numbers had already fallen well below the peak in 2015.[63]

Even if the likelihood of a threat happening (p) has been accurately measured and is known to all, some people will bet on their luck (risk prone) while others will feel they are better safe than sorry (risk averse). Among 70 people receiving treatment for opioid use disorder in a community-based centre in the US, those who were willing to make risky bets in a game of chance were also more likely to relapse to drug use.[64] When people are offered screening tests for colon, breast, or prostate cancer, and told that experts have conflicting opinions about the value of these tests, those who are more averse to ambiguity are less willing to be tested—they perceive screening to have lesser benefits and greater harms.[65,66] Differences in expert opinion can therefore put doubting patients at risk if they underestimate the benefits of screening.

Gambling with fortune carries the prospect of making gains and incurring losses, and equivalent gains and losses are not necessarily valued in the same way. Experimental tests of 'prospect theory' have found that a loss of money, for example, tends to be valued more than an equivalent gain. Because people dislike losses (e.g. of money) more than equivalent gains, they are more willing to take risks to avoid those losses.[67]

Loss aversion should favour prevention, but does not always apply to health.[4] There are at least two possible reasons. First, good health tends to be taken for granted; the unworried well do not value their health until it is lost. More insidiously, poor health, linked for example to diet, inactivity, and obesity, may come to be accepted as normal by individuals and by society, so there is no reason to do anything about it.[4] Second, better health, while clearly possible, may incur immediate costs but yield only delayed benefits (taking physical exercise, giving up smoking). For both reasons, the application of prospect theory to health and prevention needs to be probed more deeply.

Even when the evidence for a new method of prevention is scientifically clear, it will not necessarily be applied quickly (Chapter 1). The uptake of a new idea depends on the nature of the innovation (its relative advantage and complexity), on communication (personal, media), on time (to convey knowledge and persuade users), and on the social system in which implementation is carried out (who is in authority, mode of collective action).[68] Brooks and colleagues investigated the time taken by countries to adopt four new vaccines (hepatitis B, *Haemophilus influenzae* type B, Rotavirus, *Pneumococcus*) and three novel malaria interventions.[69] Among all the possibilities studied—availability, coordination, and financing of the interventions—a recommendation from the World Health Organization was the only factor consistently associated with the decision to implement sooner rather than later.

Costs and benefits of prevention: Practice

What does prevention cost today and what are the benefits? According to analyses based on the international System of Health Accounts (SHA, Box 2.2), only 3% of the US$6.7 trillion spent on health in 2017 was allocated to prevention and public health while more than 90% was spent on treatment, rehabilitation, and long-term care.[20,70] This figure varies among OECD countries, but typically lies in the range 2%–6%, depending on levels of investment and accounting methods.[20,71–73]

But this analysis does not reflect the true investment in prevention globally, for two main reasons. First, the 3% has been measured mainly in high-income (OECD) countries; the percentage is generally larger in low- and middle-income countries (Chapter 3). Second, SHA counts only spending that has direct benefits for health; it omits all spending outside the health sector that contributes indirectly to, and in turn benefits from, good health.

There have been few attempts to track spending on prevention outside the health sector. One exception is Trackfin, a system for monitoring finance for water, sanitation, and hygiene (WASH).[74,75] The benefits of WASH go well beyond health. In data collected between 2011 and 2018, 17 countries spent between 0.6% and 2.5% of gross domestic product (GDP) on WASH; 11 of these spent more on WASH than on all aspects of public health and prevention covered by SHA, including Brazil, Ghana, Kyrgyzstan, Hungary, Mali, Morocco, Nepal, and the Netherlands (Chapter 7).[74,75]

An analysis of global trends in disease incidence and mortality rates also indicates that spending is far greater than suggested by the 3%. Figure 2.2 shows that the per capita mortality and incidence rates due to 105 health conditions were mostly in decline between 1990 and 2019 (points in lower left quadrant; or left half for mortality only). About half of the proportional change in numbers of deaths from these 105 conditions can be explained by changes in case incidence (i.e. prevention; regression $R^2 = 0.56$). Per head of population, the proportional change in the incidence rate (preventing illness) was, on average, about half the proportional change in death rate (median 57%, interquartile range 26%–100%).

This analysis is consistent with (though not the same as) the finding that social, economic, and environmental factors, in combination, explain about half of the variation in the health status of populations, as judged by life expectancy (Preface).

In the past two to three decades, there have been multiple successes in reducing the incidence (prevention) of conditions with a few major, modifiable 'risk factors'—including coronary (ischaemic) heart disease (high total blood cholesterol, high blood pressure, tobacco smoking),[77,78] and vaccine preventable,[79] vector-borne[80] and other transmissible infections (prevention: illustrated by points that lie along the diagonal in Figure 2.2). In contrast, successful interventions against conditions with multiple or unpreventable causes are mostly treatments that reduce mortality, such as congenital birth defects, diarrhoeal diseases, road injuries, and upper respiratory infections (cure: points lying along the horizontal in Figure 2.2).

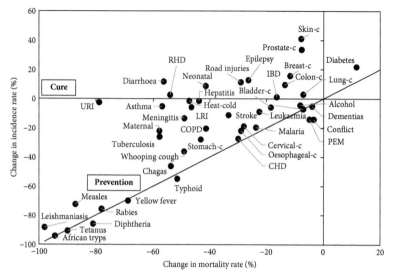

Figure 2.2 Health gains from prevention and curative treatment over three decades. Percentage change in per capita, age-standardized case incidence and mortality rates, 1990–2019, for 108 health conditions that accounted for >90% of deaths in 2019. Successful interventions against conditions with multiple or unpreventable causes are mostly due to treatments that reduce mortality e.g. congenital birth defects, diarrhoeal diseases, road injuries, and upper respiratory infections (points lie along the horizontal, slope = 0). Prevention is dominant when targeting one or a few major, modifiable 'risk factors' for illness or injury e.g. vaccine-preventable, vector-borne, and other transmissible infections (points lie along the diagonal, slope = 1). Abbreviations: African trypanosomes; Alzheimer's disease and other dementias; IBD: inflammatory bowel disease; IHD: ischaemic heart disease; COPD: chronic obstructive pulmonary disease; IBD: inflammatory bowel disease; LRI and URI: lower and upper respiratory infections; PEM: protein energy malnutrition; CHD: coronary heart disease; RHD: rheumatic heart disease; suffix -c: cancer.

Source: Data from published estimates of incidence and mortality in Institute for Health Metrics and Evaluation (IHME). GBD Compare - Viz Hub. 2020.

The exceptions to this general pattern are revealing—including malignant skin melanoma (skin-c) and typhoid (Figure 2.2). Malignant skin melanoma is mostly caused by exposure to solar irradiation, which is partly avoidable.[81,82] Among diarrhoeal diseases, which are caused by a variety of pathogens with multiple routes of transmission, the prevention of typhoid has been relatively effective because *S.* Typhi, with restricted routes of transmission ("The characteristics of prevention" above), is especially vulnerable to improvements in sanitation and hygiene.

Although the details of studies on specific health conditions may differ from the picture in Figure 2.2, it is clear that prevention has improved public health greatly over the past two to three decades, where the incidence of illness has been reduced especially through targeted interventions against major risks and hazards.

In the longer term (more than two to three decades), the success of prevention depends not just on targeted interventions but also on the circumstances of social and economic development. Figure 2.3 shows the fates of four different causes of illness and death, among many.[76] Although vaccines are available to prevent lower respiratory infections (LRIs, e.g. pneumococcal pneumonia, influenza), the short-term solutions to managing (bacterial) pneumonia are mainly antibiotic treatment and clinical care to accelerate recovery and prevent death (Figure 2.2). But over decades of development (as countries acquire a higher socio-demographic index [SDI]), the incidence of illness caused by respiratory infections has fallen alongside deaths (Figure 2.3a). Pneumonia is linked to numerous facets of poverty: the implication is that multiple effects of development are needed to lower the incidence of LRI: healthier environments (less exposure to infection), better medical services (higher vaccination rates), and healthier people (greater resistance to infection). The same is true of the multiple causes of diarrhoeal diseases, for which deaths are negligible in countries with high–middle and high SDI (Figure 2.3b).

Type 2 diabetes is largely preventable through diet and exercise but has become a global health emergency: incidence is high at all levels of SDI; only mortality has been significantly reduced, and in countries with higher levels of development (Figure 2.3c). For cancers of the trachea, bronchus, and lung, tobacco control programmes still face a huge task in reversing the adverse effects of tobacco consumption linked to social and economic development. The incidence of these cancers is highest in countries with middle and high SDI—a failure of prevention (Figure 2.3d).

Although the examples in Figure 2.3 present a mixed picture of prevention in development, social and economic advances are generally a force for better health. A 2017 study of 35 OECD countries estimated the improvements to life expectancy obtained from 10% increases in income (a gain of 2.2 months in life expectancy), primary education (3.2 months), healthier lifestyles including lower alcohol or tobacco consumption and healthier

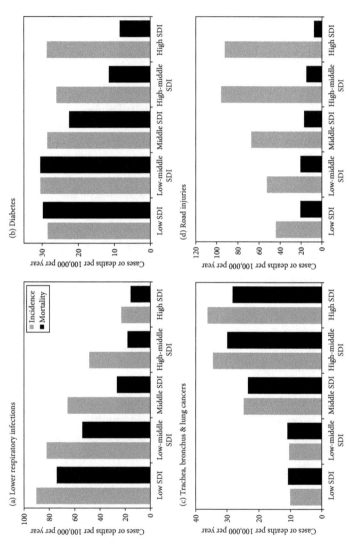

Figure 2.3 Long-term gains and losses from prevention and curative treatment worldwide: four examples using a socio-demographic index (SDI) as a measure of development running over decades: (a) Lower respiratory infections, (b) Diabetes, (c) Trachea, bronchus, and lung cancers, (d) Road injuries.

Source: Data from published estimates of incidence and mortality in Institute for Health Metrics and Evaluation (IHME). GBD Compare - Viz Hub. 2020.

diets (2.6 months), and higher levels of health spending per capita on prevention as well as treatment (3.5 months).[83]

Having identified some of the factors that keep people healthy, the next question is how to modify them. It is fortunate for the health of people living in OECD countries that income increased by 42% between 1990 and 2010, and education coverage by 44%. Such changes are only partially under the control of governments, even in wealthy countries, and the health benefits are obtained largely as side effects. Over the same period in OECD countries, healthy behaviours were adopted more and less quickly, depending on the behaviour: the prevalence of smoking dropped by 31% and the quantity of alcohol consumed by 8%, while daily vegetable consumption increased by just 2%. In sum, actions to benefit health are not easily instigated by individuals or by governments, but they become more likely when both work together (Chapter 6).

The overview of principles and practice in this chapter has laid out the problem of prevention. Chapters 3–8 investigate how the problem can be solved in six specific settings—from prevention in health services to mitigation in the face of climate change.

Summary

Most people aspire to healthy living but staying healthy and preventing illness carry a cost—counted in money, time, effort, information, trust, and willpower. The principles of prevention can be framed as a conditional, testable hypothesis: prevention is more likely to be favoured when individuals or populations can choose, given the constraints presented in any setting, a low-cost, high-efficacy method of averting a large, probable, imminent threat to health. The decisions that people make about health depend, not only on quantified options, risks, hazards, and timing, but also on the incentives, motives, powers, and values of everyone who has a stake in the outcome—individuals, governments, non-governmental organizations, businesses, and others. Data presented in this chapter suggest that more money and effort are invested in prevention today than is commonly thought, but the enormous, persistent, avoidable burden of ill health is a reason to seek ways of investing still more.

References

1. Buffet W. *2009 Annual Report*. Berkshire Hathaway Inc.; 2010. https://www. annualreports.com/HostedData/AnnualReportArchive/b/NYSE_BRK-A_ 2009.pdf (accessed 16 January 2020).
2. Centers for Disease Control and Prevention. Ten great public health achievements in the 20th century. 2013. http://medbox.iiab.me/modules/en-cdc/www. cdc.gov/about/history/tengpha.htm (accessed 16 January 2020).
3. Perloff JM. *Microeconomics*. Boston, MA: Addison-Wesley; 2012.
4. Treadwell JR, Lenert LA. Health values and prospect theory. *Medical Decision Making* 1999; *19*: 344–52.
5. Morgan MG, Kandlikar M, Risbey J, Dowlatabadi H. Why conventional tools for policy analysis are often inadequate for problems of global change. *Climatic Change* 1999; *41*: 271–81.
6. Hauck K, Smith PC. Public choice analysis of public health priority setting. In: Culyer AJ, ed. *Encyclopedia of Health Economics*. San Diego: Elsevier; 2014: 184–93.
7. Owen L, Morgan A, Fischer A, Ellis S, Hoy A, Kelly MP. The cost-effectiveness of public health interventions. *Journal of Public Health (Oxford Academic)* 2012; *34*: 37–45.
8. National Institute for Health and Care Excellence (NICE). *Hypertension in Adults: Diagnosis and Management (NG136)*. London: NICE; 2019.
9. Feikin DR, Flannery B, Hamel MJ, Stack M, Hansen PM. Vaccines for children in low- and middle-income countries. In: Black RE, Laxminarayan R, Temmerman M, Walker N, eds. *Reproductive, Maternal, Newborn, and Child Health: Disease Control Priorities*, 3rd edn (Volume 2). Washington, DC: The International Bank for Reconstruction and Development/The World Bank; 2016: Chapter 10.
10. Sambala EZ, Wiyeh AB, Ngcobo N, Machingaidze S, Wiysonge CS. New vaccine introductions in Africa before and during the decade of vaccines—Are we making progress? *Vaccine* 2019; *37*: 3290–5.
11. Burchett HE, Mounier-Jack S, Griffiths UK, et al. New vaccine adoption: Qualitative study of national decision-making processes in seven low- and middle-income countries. *Health Policy and Planning* 2012; *27*: ii5–16.
12. Mills A. Reflections on the development of health economics in low- and middle-income countries. *Proceedings of the Royal Society B* 2014; *281*: 20140451.
13. Burchett HE, Mounier-Jack S, Griffiths UK, Mills AJ. National decision-making on adopting new vaccines: A systematic review. *Health Policy Plan* 2012; *27*: ii62–76.
14. Allin S, Mossialos E, McKee M, Holland W. *Making Decisions in Public Health: A Review of Eight Countries*. Copenhagen: World Health Organization; 2004.
15. Allin S, Mossialos E, McKee M, Holland W. The Wanless report and decision-making in public health. *Journal of Public Health (Oxford Academic)* 2005; *27*: 133–4.

16. Dye C. National and international policies to mitigate disease threats. *Philosophical Transactions of the Royal Society B: Biological Sciences* 2012; *367*: 2893–900.

17. Alageel S, Gulliford MC. Health checks and cardiovascular risk factor values over six years' follow-up: Matched cohort study using electronic health records in England. *PLoS Medicine* 2019; *16*: e1002863.

18. Heneghan C, Mahtani KR. Is it time to end general health checks? *BMJ Evidence Based Medicine* 2019; *25*: 115–16.

19. Krogsboll LT, Jorgensen KJ, Gotzsche PC. General health checks in adults for reducing morbidity and mortality from disease. *Cochrane Database of Systematic Reviews* 2019; *1*: CD009009.

20. Gmeinder M, Morgan D, Mueller M. *How Much Do OECD Countries Spend on Prevention?* Paris: Organisation for Economic Co-operation and Development; 2017.

21. Baddeley M. *Behavioural Economics: A Very Short Introduction.* Oxford: Oxford University Press; 2016.

22. Hough DE. *Irrationality in Health Care: What Behavioral Economics Reveals about What We Do and Why.* Stanford: Stanford University Press; 2013.

23. Gigerenzer G. *Simply Rational. Decision Making in the Real World.* Oxford: Oxford University Press; 2015.

24. Kelly MP. Cognitive biases in public health and how economics and sociology can help overcome them. *Public Health* 2019; *169*: 163–72.

25. Rice T. The behavioral economics of health and health care. *Annual Review of Public Health* 2013; *34*: 431–47.

26. Davies NB, Krebs JR, West SA. *An Introduction to Behavioural Ecology.* Chichester: Wiley; 2012.

27. The Behavioural Insights Team. *Annual Report 2017–18.* London: Behavioural Insights Ltd; 2019.

28. Thaler R. *Misbehaving.* New York: WW Norton & Company; 2015.

29. Fuller G. *The Invisible Killer: The Rising Global Threat of Air Pollution—and How We Can Fight Back.* New York: Melville House; 2018.

30. Fuller GJ. Review of Our Lethal Air by Jonathan Mingle. New York Review of Books. 26 September 2019.

31. Greater London Authority. *Report of the London Assembly's Investigative Committee on Smoking in Public Places.* London: Greater London Authority; 2002.

32. Beckett L. Elizabeth Warren reframes mass shooting debate after Virginia Beach. The Guardian. 2 June 2019.

33. Gun Violence Archive. Gun Violence Archive 2019. 2019. https://www.gunviolencearchive.org (accessed 16 January 2021).

34. Torjesen I. Can public health strategies tackle London's rise in fatal violence? *BMJ* 2018; *361*: k1578.

35. Massey J, Sherman LW, Coupe T. Forecasting knife homicide risk from prior knife assaults in 4835 local areas of London, 2016–2018. *Cambridge Journal of Evidence-Based Policing* 2019; online 14 April.

36. Sunstein CR, Zeckhauser R. Overreaction to fearsome risks. *Environmental and Resource Economics* 2011; *48*: 435–49.
37. Fineberg HV. The paradox of disease prevention: Celebrated in principle, resisted in practice. *Journal of the American Medical Association* 2013; *310*: 85–90.
38. Levin S, Greenfield P. Monsanto ordered to pay $289m as jury rules weedkiller caused man's cancer. The Guardian. 11 August 2018.
39. International Agency for Research on Cancer (IARC). *IARC Monographs, Volume 112: Some Organophosphate Insecticides and Herbicides.* Lyon: IARC; 2015.
40. Samdal GB, Eide GE, Barth T, Williams G, Meland E. Effective behaviour change techniques for physical activity and healthy eating in overweight and obese adults; systematic review and meta-regression analyses. *International Journal of Behavioral Nutrition and Physical Activity* 2017; *14*: 42.
41. Kickbusch I, Allen L, Franz C. The commercial determinants of health. *Lancet Global Health* 2016; *4*: e895–e6.
42. McKee M, Stuckler D. Revisiting the corporate and commercial determinants of health. *American Journal of Public Health* 2018; *108*: 1167–70.
43. Adongo PB, Tabong PT, Asampong E, Ansong J, Robalo M, Adanu RM. Preparing towards preventing and containing an Ebola virus disease outbreak: What socio-cultural practices may affect containment efforts in Ghana? *PLoS Neglected Tropical Diseases* 2016; *10*: e0004852.
44. Wagner EG, Lanoix JN. Excreta disposal for rural areas and small communities. *Monograph Series of the World Health Organization* 1958; *39*: 1–182.
45. Penakalapati G, Swarthout J, Delahoy MJ, et al. Exposure to animal feces and human health: A systematic review and proposed research priorities. *Environmental Science and Technology* 2017; *51*: 11537–52.
46. Organization for Economic Co-operation and Development (OECD). *Financing Water: Investing in Sustainable Growth.* Paris: OECD; 2018.
47. World Health Organization. Diarrhoeal disease. 2017. https://www.who.int/news-room/fact-sheets/detail/diarrhoeal-disease (accessed 16 January 2021).
48. World Health Organization. Nutrition: supporting reviews. 2019. https://www.who.int/nutrition/publications/guidelines/updates_management_SAM_infantandchildren_review/en (accessed 16 January 2021).
49. Clasen T, Schmidt WP, Rabie T, Roberts I, Cairncross S. Interventions to improve water quality for preventing diarrhoea: Systematic review and meta-analysis. *BMJ* 2007; *334*: 782.
50. Clasen TF, Bostoen K, Schmidt WP, et al. Interventions to improve disposal of human excreta for preventing diarrhoea. *Cochrane Database of Systematic Reviews* 2010: CD007180.
51. Keusch GT, Walker CF, Das JK, Horton S, Habte D. Diarrheal diseases. In: Black RE, Laxminarayan R, Temmerman M, Walker N, eds. *Reproductive, Maternal, Newborn, and Child Health: Disease Control Priorities*, 3rd edn (Volume 2). Washington, DC: The International Bank for Reconstruction and Development/The World Bank; 2016: 163–86.
52. Shakya M. Phase 3 efficacy analysis of a typhoid conjugate vaccine trial in Nepal. *New England Journal of Medicine* 2019; *381*: 2209–18.

53. Nalin DR, Cash RA. 50 years of oral rehydration therapy: The solution is still simple. *Lancet* 2018; *392*: 536–8.
54. Hutton G, Chase C. Water supply, sanitation, and hygiene. In: Mock CN, Nugent R, Kobusingye O, Smith KR, eds. *Injury Prevention and Environmental Health*. Washington, DC: World Bank; 2017: 171–98.
55. Weirich P. Time preference. 2008. https://www.encyclopedia.com/social-sciences/applied-and-social-sciences-magazines/time-preference (accessed 16 January 2021).
56. Cohen JD, Ericson KM, Laibson D, White JM. Measuring time preferences. *NBER Working Paper No. 22455* 2019.
57. Hauck K, Smith PC. *The Politics of Priority Setting in Health: A Political Economy Perspective*. Washington DC: Center for Global Development; 2015.
58. Jamison D, Gelband H, Horton S, et al. DCP3: Disease Control Priorities. 2018. http://dcp-3.org (accessed 7 January 2021).
59. Bernoulli D. Exposition of a new theory on the measurement of risk. *Econometrica* 1954; *22*: 23–36.
60. Oltedal S, Moen B-E, Klempe H, Rundmo T. *Explaining Risk Perception. An Evaluation of Cultural Theory*. Trondheim: Norwegian University of Science and Technology; 2004.
61. Ropeik D. The psychology of risk perception. *Harvard Mental Health Letter* 2011; (June).
62. Carman KG, Kooreman P. Probability perceptions and preventive health care. *Journal of Risk and Uncertainty* 2014; *49*: 43–71.
63. United Nations High Commissioner for Refugees (UNHCR). *Desperate Journeys. Refugees and Migrants Arriving in Europe and at Europe's Borders. January–December 2018*. Geneva: UNHCR; 2019.
64. Konova AB, Lopez-Guzman S, Urmanche A, et al. Computational markers of risky decision-making for identification of temporal windows of vulnerability to opioid use in a real-world clinical setting. *JAMA Psychiatry* 2019; *77*: 368–77.
65. Han PK, Kobrin SC, Klein WM, Davis WW, Stefanek M, Taplin SH. Perceived ambiguity about screening mammography recommendations: Association with future mammography uptake and perceptions. *Cancer Epidemiology, Biomarkers and Prevention* 2007; *16*: 458–66.
66. Han PK, Williams AE, Haskins A, et al. Individual differences in aversion to ambiguity regarding medical tests and treatments: Association with cancer screening cognitions. *Cancer Epidemiology, Biomarkers and Prevention* 2014; *23*: 2916–23.
67. Kahneman D, Tversky A. Prospect theory: An analysis of decision under risk. *Econometrica* 1979; *47*: 263–91.
68. Rogers EM. *Diffusion of Innovations*. 5th edn. New York: Free Press; 2003.
69. Brooks A, Smith TA, de Savigny D, Lengeler C. Implementing new health interventions in developing countries: Why do we lose a decade or more? *BioMed Central Public Health* 2012; *12*: 683.
70. Office for National Statistics. UK Health Accounts: 2016. 2016. https://www.ons.gov.uk/peoplepopulationandcommunity/healthandsocialcare/

healthcaresystem/bulletins/ukhealthaccounts/2016#total-healthcare-expenditure-by-function-and-provider.

71. Fenina A, Geffroy Y, Minc C, Renaud T, Sarlon E, Sermet C. *Les Dépenses de Prévention et les Dépenses de Soins par Pathologie en France*. Paris: DREES; 2006.

72. Rechel B. Funding for public health in Europe in decline? *Health Policy* 2019; *123*: 21–6.

73. Watkins DA, Nugent R, Saxenian H, et al. Intersectoral Policy Priorities for Health. In: Jamison DT, Gelband H, Horton, S, et al., eds. *Disease Control Priorities: Improving Health and Reducing Poverty*. Washington, DC: The International Bank for Reconstruction and Development/The World Bank; 2017.

74. UN-Water and World Health Organization. *TrackFin Initiative: Tracking Financing to Sanitation, Hygiene and Drinking-Water at the national level*. Geneva: World Health Organization; 2015.

75. World Health Organization and UN-Water. *UN-Water Global Analysis and Assessment of Sanitation and Drinking-Water (GLAAS) 2019 Report: National Systems to Support Drinking-Water, Sanitation and Hygiene—Global Status Report 2019*. Geneva: World Health Organization; 2019.

76. Institute for Health Metrics and Evaluation (IHME). *GBD Compare—Viz Hub*. 2020. https://vizhub.healthdata.org/gbd-compare (accessed 16 January 2021).

77. Ford ES, Capewell S. Proportion of the decline in cardiovascular mortality disease due to prevention versus treatment: Public health versus clinical care. *Annual Review of Public Health* 2011; *32*: 5–22.

78. Ezzati M, Obermeyer Z, Tzoulaki I, Mayosi BM, Elliott P, Leon DA. Contributions of risk factors and medical care to cardiovascular mortality trends. *Nature Reviews Cardiology* 2015; *12*: 508–30.

79. Piot P, Larson HJ, O'Brien KL, et al. Immunization: vital progress, unfinished agenda. *Nature* 2019; *575*: 119–29.

80. World Health Organization. *World Malaria Report*. Geneva: World Health Organization; 2018.

81. Sample A, He YY. Mechanisms and prevention of UV-induced melanoma. *Photodermatol Photoimmunol Photomed* 2018; *34*: 13–24.

82. Parkin DM, Mesher D, Sasieni P. 13. Cancers attributable to solar (ultraviolet) radiation exposure in the UK in 2010. *British Journal of Cancer* 2011; *105*: S66–9.

83. Organization for Economic Cooperation and Development (OECD). *Health at a Glance 2017: OECD Indicators*. Paris: OECD; 2017.

3
The affordable dream

Ring-fence the prevention budget.
Derek Bell (Royal College of Physicians of Edinburgh, 2019)[1]

Universal Health Coverage (UHC) is Amartya Sen's 'affordable dream'.[2] UHC means that everyone has access to the health services they need—preventing as well as treating illness—without risk of financial hardship. UHC contributes to equity as a major goal of sustainable development—'to ensure that no one is left behind'.[3] Because health promotion and disease prevention address both the immediate and underlying causes of illness, they compete for resources within the health sector and with other sectors of government. In both competitions, prevention starts from a position of disadvantage.

Prevention and universal health coverage

Sen's focus was on the low-income countries that are furthest away from achieving UHC today. He made his case by pointing to the low costs and large, equitable benefits of public health services that are on show in Costa Rica, Kerala (India), Rwanda, Sri Lanka, and Thailand. He then compared them with overpriced and inefficient private health care in these countries and elsewhere.

To the extent that public health services have the various qualities described by Sen, they are not yet expressed persuasively enough to put most countries on track to achieve UHC. Based on recent trends, only 40%–60% of people worldwide will have access to essential health services by 2030, the date set to achieve the United Nations Sustainable Development Goals (SDGs).[4] To meet targets for the health-related SDGs, centred on UHC (target 3.8), the governments of low- and middle-income countries will

The Great Health Dilemma. Christopher Dye, Oxford University Press. © Oxford University Press 2021.
DOI: 10.1093/oso/9780198853824.003.0003

have to markedly increase public spending on health—by a factor of two or three times.[5,6]

To increase expenditure on prevention, as a part of the drive towards UHC, is a big challenge because, even when more money is spent on health, there is a strong inclination, everywhere in the world, to fund clinical services first.[7] Clinical medicine is the default in health care. However, the present inward-looking focus on healthcare services, as the centrepiece of health under the SDGs, threatens to limit the opportunities for prevention that come from engagement with the broader ambitions of social, economic, and environmental development.

The recommitment to primary health care, following the fortieth anniversary of the 1978 Alma Ata Declaration,[8] has the potential to support prevention because primary care is the front line for public health and community participation.[9-11] However, prevention is not top priority even in primary care, where spending is driven mostly by outpatient and home-based consultations and by the cost of medicines.[12] Health promotion in primary care, including prevention and 'social prescribing' (community services that support health and welfare) are works in progress, with an underdeveloped evidence base on who is most likely to benefit and what type of interventions are most effective.[13-17]

In Britain's post-1945 combat against William Beveridge's 'five giants'— want, ignorance, disease, squalor, and idleness (in other words, income, education, health, housing, and employment), the National Health Service was just one part of a vision of social reconstruction and progress. Beveridge's vision was of a nation with a common purpose: 'Freedom from want cannot be forced on a democracy or given to a democracy. It must be won by them. Winning it needs ... a sense of national unity.'[18]

Today, that vision of health as integral to social and economic progress is framed in the way health contributes to, and benefits from, the SDGs through action on poverty (SDG 1), education (SDG 4), sustainable cities and communities (SDG 11), and decent work and economic growth (SDG 8), among others.[7,11]

In England, the question of how to link health and well-being has frequently been revisited over the eight decades since World War II. The 2004 Wanless report on *Securing Good Health for the Whole Population*[19] drew conclusions that are still relevant now, and which apply far beyond the English context:

Numerous policy statements and initiatives in the field of public health have not resulted in a rebalancing of policy away from health care (a 'national sickness service') to health (a 'national health service'). This will not happen until there is a realignment of incentives in the system to focus on reducing the burden of disease and tackling the key lifestyle and environmental risks. Reducing the burden of disease … needs a clear articulation of the priorities for action with accountabilities defined both within and outside of the National Health Service.

Taking up the challenge, this chapter explores ways to realign the incentives for prevention within health services. The next section is a preface to that discussion, spelling out the problem of prevention in more detail.

Prevention is ancillary to cure

From the disadvantaged perspective of prevention, national healthcare services make an unmatchable proposition: whatever kind of illness or injury befalls a person, the health service offers some form of treatment. In contrast, besides general[19] and even statutory[20] guidance on maintaining good health, including health-supporting policies such as national education services, there is no similarly comprehensive offer for prevention.

As nations become wealthier, they spend more on health,[21] but spending on medical treatment apparently increases more quickly than spending on prevention. Consequently, as health budgets grow larger over years and decades, the proportion of these budgets allocated to prevention declines, falling from as much as 30% in some low-income countries to around 3% in high-income Organisation for Economic Co-operation and Development (OECD) countries (Figure 3.1; Chapter 2).[22]

In the short term, too, prevention is invariably among the first casualties of economic hardship. After the 2007–08 financial crisis, the fall in Gross Domestic Product (GDP) growth in OECD countries was followed by a bigger reduction in spending on prevention than on health in total (Figure 3.2).[22–24] Prevention and public health were particularly vulnerable to funding cuts in England, France, Moldova, the Netherlands, and Slovenia.[23,25,26]

In England, the disadvantage faced by prevention and public health has persisted well beyond the 2007–08 economic downturn: between 2015/16 and 2019/20, spending overall on the National Health Service grew

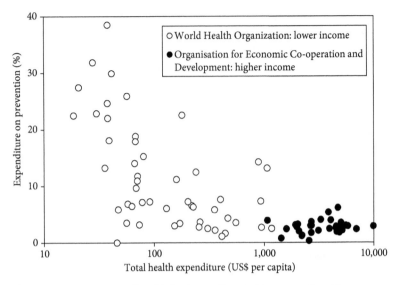

Figure 3.1 Percentage of health budgets allocated to prevention. The percentage is greater in higher-income countries that spend more on health (Organisation for Economic Co-operation and Development [OECD] data, each filled circle represents a country) than in lower-income countries that spend less on health (World Health Organization [WHO] data, open circles).

Source: Data from OECD. Health expenditure and financing. 2020. https://stats.oecd.org/ Index.aspx?DataSetCode=SHA; World Health Organization. Global Health Expenditure Database. 2020. https://apps.who.int/nha/database.

by 8% per person in real terms and yet the public health grant was cut by 23%.[27,28] A 2018 United Kingdom government green paper entitled 'Prevention Is Better than Cure'[29] illuminated the chasm between political rhetoric and funding reality. In the lead up to the 2019 general election, political debate was dominated by promises to build and renovate hospitals, which are judged to hold greater popular appeal than helping people stay healthy and well.[29-31] During the COVID-19 pandemic in 2020, hospital services were given priority. During August 2020, the service responsible for all aspects of public health and prevention (including infectious and non-communicable diseases), Public Health England, was disbanded and replaced by a new National Institute for Health Protection (NIPH). The NIPH is oriented towards a centrally controlled pandemic and emergency response system, with a strong emphasis on private contracting, rather than a locally driven, broad-based, publicly funded response to prevention

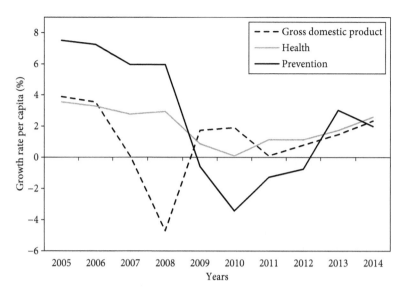

Figure 3.2 Finance for prevention in Organisation for Economic Co-operation and Development (OECD) countries was disproportionately affected by the 2007–08 financial crisis: the fall in gross domestic product (GDP) growth (dashed line) was followed by a bigger reduction in spending on prevention (black line) than on health in total (grey line). But growth in all three quantities had recovered by 2014–15.

Adapted with permission from Gmeinder M., Morgan D., Mueller M. (2017). How much do OECD countries spend on prevention?, *OECD Health Working Papers*, Paris, France: OECD Publishing.

(including preparedness), integrated into the national healthcare system.[32] The NIPH is not due to be fully functional until 2021, but initial signs (in August 2020) do not point to rapid reinvestment in prevention and public health (Box 2.2), supporting programmes for the control of obesity; drug, alcohol, and tobacco use; and immunization and the containment of other infectious diseases.[33]

The pressure on prevention is not unique to the UK. Budgets for prevention and public health are routinely under assault around the world. In the United States, public health spending per person in real terms rose from $39 in 1960 to $281 in 2008 but has fallen steadily since then. This public health disadvantage appears to have deeper roots than the 2007–08 financial crisis because public health's share of total health expenditure in the US has been in decline since 2002.[34]

The squeeze on prevention and public health budgets is also visible in state and local governments in the US, which are the main source of public health dollars. The rising cost of medical care in California has put enormous pressure on funds for other services including public education, public health, food and housing assistance, and income support. In 2007, spending on public health, the environment, and social services was $1.22 for every dollar spent on medical care, but had fallen to just $0.68 by 2018.[35]

Public health budgets are difficult to defend, in part because the adverse effects of cuts are hard to measure precisely. Ever since the 2007–08 financial crisis, public service professionals have argued that austerity—imposed by tightening the reins on government spending—is a killer. In England, two research studies concluded that the failure to maintain investment in health and social care (including the prevention of unhealthy behaviours such as alcohol and tobacco consumption, poor diet, and low physical activity) caused more than 100,000 preventable deaths between 2012 and 2017.[36,37] These estimates have been accompanied by observations on reductions in life expectancy at birth: most conspicuously, women living in the most deprived areas of England lost nearly 100 days of life expectancy between 2012–14 and 2015–17, in contrast to an increase of 84 days in the least deprived areas.[38,39] In 2019, the UN Special Rapporteur on extreme poverty and human rights reported that 'policies of austerity introduced in 2010 continue largely unabated, despite the tragic social consequences.'[40]

Doubtful data and differences of expert opinion are impediments to public motivation and political action. In the UK, some of the evidence surrounding the causes and numbers of deaths was anecdotal, circumstantial, and inconsistent, and the impact of austerity was openly disputed.[41–45] Public disagreement among experts loosens the reins on government accountability.

In the face of such obstacles, the best way to promote prevention and public health is by following the path laid out by Wanless—focusing on the constraints and the incentives, and mindful of the difficulties.[19] Drawing on the principles in Chapter 2, the rest of this chapter proposes five ways to do this. The suggestions are illustrative, not exhaustive.

Protecting the budget for prevention

Taken at face value, the question of whether prevention is better than cure suggests that there is a simple choice between the two. In the context of

health services, however, there is a constraint on choice that puts prevention at a disadvantage. Clinical care is an indispensable safety net: resources
are unlikely to be shifted from treatment to prevention until treatment becomes unnecessary.

For example, most lung cancers are preventable and could be avoided
through tobacco control, using measures including price increases through
taxation and advertising bans, plus blank or graphic cigarette packaging,
among other ways to demonstrate the dangers of smoking. But all these
measures are supplementary to the treatment of lung cancers, which will
continue until there are none left to treat (Chapter 6).

Consequently, prevention needs additional, protected funding, even if
costs or cost-benefit ratios favour prevention over cure.[1,7] Recognizing this
fact in 2002, Thailand ring-fenced 20% of its UHC budget for prevention
and health promotion.[7] Some European countries, anticipating the growing
cost of medical care in ageing populations, have followed suit: Latvia, Italy,
and France have expanded their programmes of prevention and health promotion. The 1998 Austrian Health Promotion Fund and Germany's 2017
Preventive Health Care Act give statutory force to prevention, placing ob-
ligations on private as well as public health care institutions to carry out
routine health checks and vaccination programmes, among other responsi-
bilities.[46] Finland offers services for prevention and promotion mostly free
of charge, and they are widely used. But hospital outpatient care, including
laboratory tests and scans, requires users to pay, up to a maximum set by
central government (above which this care too is free of charge). The UK
government, in contrast, has declined to protect public health budgets for
the foreseeable future, despite calls from public health professionals (one of
whom is quoted at the chapter head).[1,47]

All these initiatives must be judged by their performance in practice.
Irrespective of their success, they illustrate the range of options available
to protect or enhance financing for prevention––if there is a will to do so.
Too little is known about the circumstances under which governments are
motivated to express that will. But local details matter: Colombia created a
dedicated budget for prevention in the 1990s, separated from the budget
for medical treatment. That dedicated budget has always been under pressure, not just because of the usual preference for treatment over prevention, but also because municipal governments are not trusted to administer
funds for social insurance schemes.[7] India's drive to achieve UHC by 2030 is
partly through investment in much-needed primary health centres across
the country. But a parallel and popular health insurance scheme provides

financial protection for hospital care only, pushing public spending towards treatment and away from prevention.[48]

In California, state policymakers see no economic advantage in cutting healthcare spending through prevention because, by saving money on medical treatment, they would forfeit matching federal funds.[35] More generally, California government agencies, employers, and hospitals could improve the health of the population, and provide a larger health return on investment, by pooling their resources into 'wellness funds', as other cities and communities in the US have done. But the prevailing disincentives in California disfavour collaboration.[35]

Bounty in the eye of the beholder

Whether prevention is worth the investment depends, in part, on the perceived value of its benefits. The United States Prevention and Public Health Fund, established in 2010 with a 10-year budget of US$15 billion, is the nation's first mandatory investment mechanism for public health and prevention. The Fund has attracted controversy.[49] Critics have argued that it is too costly alongside large federal budget deficits; it has also been seen by Congress as a way of paying for the repeal of President Barack Obama's Patient Protection and Affordable Care Act (Obamacare). The task for advocates of the Fund is to highlight the attributes that appeal to different political constituencies, without diminishing its effectiveness or distorting the facts. Republican lawmakers, like conservatives everywhere, favour cost reduction and small government. They want to know how the Fund will help to contain healthcare costs and how it encourages individuals to take responsibility for their own health. Democrats, on the other hand, want to know how the Fund will help widen access to health care and reduce inequalities.

Perceptions of the value of prevention can be grounded in health metrics.[50] Once a metric has been agreed and adopted, it can be used to set benchmarks and targets, and embedded in routine practice. There is (slowly) mounting pressure to replace GDP with a measure of economic welfare that better serves the age of sustainable development. GDP essentially measures monetary transactions at their market prices, whether or not those transactions are good or bad for human well-being. Commodities that have value but no market price are excluded. Among the exclusions are some of the key ingredients of social (equality, welfare, well-being) and natural capital (clean air and water, nutritious food, biodiversity, public spaces) that underpin public health.

Resistance to the idea of modifying GDP rests, in part, on the fact that GDP was devised to measure economic activity, not welfare. Defenders of GDP suggest that other indices should be used to quantify welfare or well-being. The alternatives include the Human Development Index,[51] the Gross National Happiness Index,[52,53] the Social Progress Index,[54] the OECD well-being framework,[55] and the Inclusive Wealth Index.[56,57] Some are gaining traction, slowly. In New Zealand's 2019 'well-being budget', all new spending must support five well-being goals: fostering mental health, reducing child poverty, supporting indigenous peoples, creating a sustainable low-carbon economy, and thriving in the digital age.[58]

The UK Office of National Statistics publishes measures of personal well-being that look beyond GDP to health, personal relationships, education and skills, and the environment. In that context, the UK government has begun to explore improved measures of population health—a composite Health Index for England. Its stated purpose is to frame health as a primary national asset, contributing both to the economy and to the happiness of the population.[59] The index would support prevention by including measures, not just of health outcomes, but also of modifiable risk factors and the social determinants of health. These intentions must, however, be judged against a background of falling investment in public health.

Optimal prevention

Data gathered via the international System of Health Accounts (SHA) show that the proportion of national health budgets allocated to prevention and public health is more or less independent of national wealth (Chapter 2).[22] But, however much is spent, better results will be obtained when the money is spent more efficiently.

Given the general preference for efficiency, a surprisingly large fraction of prevention budgets are allocated to 'healthy condition monitoring'(HCM, health check-ups)—an average of 44% in OECD countries in 2015 (Chapter 2). HCM may be applied to the whole population, or to specific conditions (e.g. pregnancy), specific age groups (e.g. children) or certain health domains, such as dental checks—even though this form of primary prevention is not usually judged to be cost-effective.[22,60,61] One assessment found that health checks of the general population have little or no effect on the number of deaths from all causes, or deaths specifically from cancer and cardiovascular disease.[61] Some health checks also require potentially harmful and invasive tests, increasing the costs in relation to the benefits.

One way to improve value for money is by identifying sub-groups of individuals who are known to be at relatively high risk of ill health. Monitoring during pregnancy is an example: although health checks in pregnancy are not generally needed, they are recommended for women who suffer from hypertension. High blood pressure during pregnancy carries risks for the mother and for the developing foetus. Focusing on women at risk is more efficient, and the efficiency can be increased in some settings by allowing women to monitor their own blood pressure at home. This reduces the frequency of hospital visits, and saves money without compromising on health.[62]

Similarly, screening for early signs of cancer in sub-populations at relatively high risk, including breast, cervical, and colorectal cancers, is cost-effective against standard benchmarks.[63] In the Republic of Korea, increased funding for early cancer detection has markedly pushed up the overall budget for prevention and public health since 2003 (Figure 3.3).

New options for prevention are bound to be revealed by deeper investigation, but prevention research is generally underfunded. In cancer care, there have been relatively few economic evaluations of primary prevention (averting disease) compared with secondary and tertiary prevention (earlier or later disease detection and treatment).[63-65] A wide-ranging review of US research, covering more than 11,000 projects between 2012 and 2017, found that only a quarter (26%) looked at preventive methods for leading causes of death—including cancer, heart disease, and stroke—even though these conditions are associated with nearly three-quarters of all deaths in the country.[66] In addition, far more money is invested in drug discovery than in vaccine development. A stronger case for prevention will rest on understanding the incentives for investment by private donors, governments, health agencies, and pharmaceutical companies (Chapter 4).

Prevention on demand

Vaccine hesitancy, and even hostility, are reminders that prevention depends on public demand as well as health service supply (Chapter 4). The factors that affect demand for preventive methods, vaccination, and others, are less well studied than the factors that affect supply.

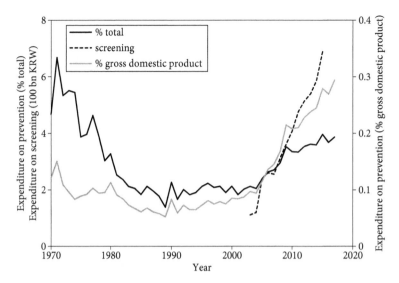

Figure 3.3 Protecting and enhancing the budget for prevention within health services, Republic of Korea. Expenditure on prevention, as a percentage of all health spending (black line), declined between 1970 and 2003, in line with the pattern in Figure 3.1. Since 2003, Korea has increased spending on early cancer detection (secondary prevention, dashed line), roughly doubling the share of total health spending on prevention from 2% to 4% (black line) and pushing up total expenditure on prevention as a percentage of gross domestic product (grey line).

Source: Data from Gmeinder M., Morgan D., Mueller M. (2017). How much do OECD countries spend on prevention?, OECD Health Working Papers, Paris, France: OECD Publishing.

The case studies that have been done show that some of the determinants of demand are generally applicable, while others depend on local details. In general, the public uptake of preventive care offered by health services, such as HCM and cancer screening, is higher among wealthier and well-educated people.[67,68] But even for health-conscious, well-informed consumers, supply must meet demand: in Italy, the non-monetary costs of (free) screening for breast and cervical cancer have been deterrents to use, including difficulties of access for women living in rural areas, and long waiting times at underequipped health facilities.[69]

Locally, the details of health insurance policies influence how prevention and treatment services for breast and cervical cancer are used. Insurance for medical treatment could, in principle, present a moral hazard, discouraging prevention. However, some research has found that insurance for treatment can stimulate rather than depress demand for prevention. The likely explanation is that screening (early detection) is thought to be worthwhile when insurance covers treatment costs in the event of a positive diagnosis.[67]

Likewise, workplace health promotion encourages prevention in some settings,[70] but outcomes depend on the way such programmes are implemented. Health policies should not, for instance, save medical costs to employers by shifting those costs to vulnerable employees, a danger that emerged as an unintended consequence of the US Affordable Care Act.[71,72] Other methods of stimulating demand for prevention that vary in success among settings include cash transfers (to relieve financial hardship, support education, assist with birth registration),[73] membership of labour unions (to facilitate the use of employee cancer screening programmes),[74] and advocacy for public health by citizens' interest groups.[75]

Public information and education campaigns (from within the health sector) do have some influence, but facts have greater force when coupled with incentives (often outside the control of the health sector). With regard to healthy eating, for example, these include taxes on sugary drinks and snacks, obligatory food reformulation, food labelling, and food subsidies. When people become aware of the harms of unhealthy eating, they often want to help to change their diets. The form of that help is a matter of debate: laws and regulations that reduce the consumption of harmful products—salt, sugar, trans fat, and tobacco—have to be forged in public discussion about the pros and cons of government intervention (Chapter 6).[76]

Prevention in all policies

The movement to put Health in All Policies (HiAP)—making health part of decision making across the whole of government—preceded, but has become integral to, the SDG agenda.[77] Initiatives in other sectors of government that promote and benefit from good health are largely preventive. In other words, HiAP is, by and large, prevention in all policies.

From the perspective of prevention, the SDGs constitute an expanded health system, linking health with agriculture, education, employment, energy, environment, finance, trade, transport, and urban planning, potentially with multiple mutual benefits (not neglecting possible conflicts).[78–80] SDG 3, the principal health goal, fosters prevention by setting targets—to cut deaths from road traffic injuries (3.6) and from air, water, and soil pollution (3.9)—that require actions beyond the remit of national health services.[81] That sets a research agenda for prevention too: for example, to evaluate the full costs and benefits of transport policies, going beyond injuries and emissions, and embracing other advantages such as increased physical activity.[82] Transport policies contribute to at least 12 of the 17 SDGs.[83]

Among low- and middle-income countries, Iran, Thailand, and Vietnam have led the way in placing health in all government policies.[84] The benefits are visible in health data collected across multiple sectors with presidential oversight (Iran); in the broader compass of health impact assessments, including biomass power plant projects, patents on medicines, coal mining, and industrial estate development (Thailand); and in reducing road traffic deaths through helmet laws (Vietnam).[84,85]

Prevention and public health stand to benefit greatly when they are given broad ministerial support.[86] But the reasons why Iran, Thailand, and Vietnam have chosen to do this where others have not, and whether those reasons are transferrable to other countries, are also topics for the prevention research agenda.

Summary

Prevention is integral to achieving health equity and Universal Health Coverage. And yet prevention is a healthcare orphan: it is not usually a priority in the health sector or in any other sector of government. This chapter suggests five ways to redress that disadvantage: give prevention and public health budgets that are separate and protected from medical services, based on demonstrated benefits; define the goals of prevention in collaboration with, and considering the objectives and values held by, those who make the decisions; reassess the value for money provided by preventive methods that presently command large budgets, such as 'healthy condition monitoring'; stimulate latent public demand for prevention by improving access to screening programmes, calibrating health insurance to favour prevention, and through workplace health promotion schemes, among others; and improve the appeal of prevention across the whole of government (beyond the health sector), using evidence to reinforce the long-standing goal of putting Health in All Policies.

References

1. Smith A. 'Ring-fence the prevention budget' warns top Doctor. *PharmaTimes Media Ltd*. 2019.
2. Sen A. Universal health care: The affordable dream. *Harvard Public Health Review* 2015; 4: 1–8.
3. United Nations. *The Sustainable Development Goals Report*. New York: United Nations; 2018.
4. World Health Organization. *Primary Health Care on the Road to Universal Health Coverage. 2019 Global Monitoring Report*. Geneva: World Health Organization; 2019.
5. Stenberg K, Hanssen O, Edejer TT, et al. Financing transformative health systems towards achievement of the health Sustainable Development Goals: A model for projected resource needs in 67 low-income and middle-income countries. *Lancet Global Health* 2017; 5: e875–e87.
6. Stenberg K. Guide posts for investment in primary health care and projected resource needs in 67 low-income and middle-income countries: A modelling study. *Lancet Global Health* 2019; 7: E1500–E1510.
7. Schmidt H, Gostin LO, Emanuel EJ. Public health, universal health coverage, and Sustainable Development Goals: Can they coexist? *Lancet* 2015; 386: 928–30.
8. World Health Organization and the United Nations Children's Fund (UNICEF). *Report of the Global Conference on Primary Health Care: From Alma-Ata towards Universal Health Coverage and the Sustainable Development Goals*. Geneva: World Health Organization; 2018.
9. Galea S, Kruk ME. Forty years after Alma-Ata: At the intersection of primary care and population health. *Milbank Quarterly* 2019; 97: 383–6.
10. Sumriddetchkajorn K, Shimazaki K, Ono T, Kusaba T, Sato K, Kobayashi N. Universal health coverage and primary care, Thailand. *Bulletin of the World Health Organization* 2019; 97: 415–22.
11. Sanders D, Nandi S, Labonte R, Vance C, Van Damme W. From primary health care to universal health coverage—One step forward and two steps back. *Lancet* 2019; 394: 619–21.
12. World Health Organization. *Public Spending on Health: A Closer Look at Global Trends*. Geneva: World Health Organization; 2018.
13. Peckham S, Hann A, Kendall S, Gillam S. Health promotion and disease prevention in general practice and primary care: A scoping study. *Primary Health Care Research and Development* 2017; 18: 529–40.
14. Drinkwater C, Wildman J, Moffatt S. Social prescribing. *BMJ* 2019; 364: l1285.
15. Pescheny JV, Randhawa G, Pappas Y. The impact of social prescribing services on service users: A systematic review of the evidence. *European Journal of Public Health* 2020; 30: 664–73.
16. Peckham S, Hann A, Kendall S, Gillam S. Health promotion and disease prevention in general practice and primary care: A scoping study. *Primary Health Care Research & Development* 2017; 18: 529–40.

17. Bickerdike L, Booth A, Wilson PM, Farley K, Wright K. Social prescribing: Less rhetoric and more reality. A systematic review of the evidence. *BMJ Open* 2017; *7*: e013384.
18. Beveridge W. *Social Insurance and Allied Services*. London: Her Majesty's Stationery Office; 1942.
19. Wanless D. *Securing Good Health for the Whole Population*. London: Her Majesty's Stationery Office; 2004.
20. Welsh Government. *Shared Purpose: Shared Future. Statutory Guidance on the Well-Being of Future Generations (Wales) Act 2015*. Cardiff: Welsh Government; 2015.
21. World Health Organization. *New Perspectives on Global Health Spending for Universal Health Coverage*. Geneva: World Health Organization; 2017.
22. Gmeinder M, Morgan D, Mueller M. *How Much Do OECD Countries Spend on Prevention?* Paris: Organisation for Economic Co-operation and Development; 2017.
23. Rechel B. Funding for public health in Europe in decline? *Health Policy* 2019; *123*: 21–6.
24. Organisation for Economic Co-operation and Development (OECD). *Health at a Glance 2017: OECD Indicators*. Paris: OECD; 2017.
25. Organisation for Economic Co-operation and Development (OECD). Health expenditure and financing. 2020. https://stats.oecd.org/Index.aspx?DataSetCode=SHA (accessed 7 January 2021).
26. World Health Organization. Global Health Expenditure Database. 2020. https://apps.who.int/nha/database (accessed 7 January 2021).
27. Elwell-Sutton T, Tinson A, Greszczuk C, et al. *Creating Healthy Lives. A Whole-Government Approach to Long-Term Investment in the Nation's Health*. London: The Health Foundation; 2019.
28. British Medical Association. *Funding for Ill-Health Prevention and Public Health in the UK*. London: British Medical Association; 2017.
29. Department of Health and Social Care. *Prevention Is Better than Cure: Our Vision to Help You Live Well for Longer*. London: Department of Health and Social Care; 2018.
30. Buck D, Baylis A, Dougall D, Robertson R. *A Vision for Population Health: Towards a Healthier Future*. London: The King's Fund; 2018.
31. Rae M, Middleton J. Health, wellbeing, and care should be top of everyone's political agenda. *BMJ* 2019; *367*: l6503.
32. HM Government. Government creates new National Institute for Health Protection. 2020. https://www.gov.uk/government/news/government-creates-new-national-institute-for-health-protection (accessed 7 January 2021).
33. Royal Society of Public Health. Questions over the future of prevention hang over the launch of the Government's plans for public health. 2020. https://www.rsph.org.uk/about-us/news/questions-over-the-future-of-prevention-hang-over-the-launch-of-the-government-s-plans-for-public-health.html (accessed 7 January 2021).
34. Himmelstein DU, Woolhandler S. Public health's falling share of US health spending. *American Journal of Public Health* 2016; *106*: 56–7.

35. Brownlee S, Saini V, Garber J. *California's Health Care Paradox: Too Much Health Care Spending May Lead to Poor Community Health*. Brookline, MA: The Lown Institute; 2019.

36. Watkins J, Wulaningsih W, Da Zhou C, et al. Effects of health and social care spending constraints on mortality in England: A time trend analysis. *BMJ Open* 2017; 7: e017722.

37. Hochlaf D, Quilter-Pinner H, Kibasi T. *Ending the Blame Game: The Case for a New Approach to Public Health and Prevention*. London: Institute for Public Policy Research; 2019.

38. Office for National Statistics. *Health State Life Expectancies by National Deprivation Deciles, England and Wales: 2015 to 2017*. London: Office for National Statistics; 2019.

39. Marmot M, Allen J, Boyce T, Goldblatt P, Morrison J. *Health Equity in England: The Marmot Review 10 Years on*. London: Institute of Health Equity; 2020.

40. Alston P. *Visit to the United Kingdom of Great Britain and Northern Ireland. Report of the Special Rapporteur on Extreme Poverty and Human Rights*. New York: United Nations Human Rights Council; 2019.

41. McDermid V. Is austerity linked to 120,000 unnecessary deaths? 2018. https://fullfact.org/health/austerity-120000-unnecessary-deaths (accessed 7 January 2021).

42. Quilter-Pinner H, Hochlaf D. *Austerity: There Is an Alternative and the UK can Afford to Deliver It*. London: Institute for Public Policy Research; 2019.

43. Raleigh VS. *Trends in Life Expectancy in EU and Other OECD Countries: Why Are Improvements Slowing?* Paris: Organisation for Economic Co-operation and Development; 2019.

44. Sachs J. Paul Krugman has got it wrong on austerity. The Guardian. 6 January 2015.

45. Krugman P. The case for cuts was a lie. Why does Britain still believe it? The austerity delusion. The Guardian. 29 April 2015.

46. European Commission. *Joint Report on Health Care and Long-Term Care Systems & Fiscal Sustainability. Country Documents 2019 Update*. Luxembourg: Publications Office of the European Union; 2019.

47. Iacobucci G. Government dismisses call to ringfence public health budgets. *BMJ* 2018; 360: k891.

48. Brundtland GH. India's health reforms: The need for balance. *Lancet* 2018; 392: 1174–5.

49. Fraser MR. A brief history of the prevention and public health fund: Implications for public health advocates. *American Journal of Public Health* 2019; 109: 572–7.

50. Kruk ME, Ataguba JE, Akweongo P. The universal health coverage ambition faces a critical test. *Lancet* 2020; 396, 17 October.

51. United Nations Development Programme. Human Development Index (HDI). 2019. http://hdr.undp.org/en/content/human-development-index-hdi (accessed 7 January 2021).

52. Oxford Poverty & Human Development Initiative (OPHI). Bhutan's Gross National Happiness Index. 2019. https://ophi.org.uk/policy/gross-national-happiness-index (accessed 7 January 2021).

53. Global Council for Happiness and Wellbeing. *Global Happiness and Wellbeing Policy Report*. New York: Sustainable Development Solutions Network; 2019.

54. The Social Progress Imperative. 2019 Social Progress Index. 2019. https://www.socialprogress.org (accessed 7 January 2021).

55. OECD. Measuring well-being and progress: Well-being research. 2019. https://www.oecd.org/statistics/measuring-well-being-and-progress.htm (accessed 7 January 2021).

56. UN Environment. *The Inclusive Wealth Report (IWR)*. Nairobi: UN Environment; 2018.

57. Dasgupta P. *The Economics of Biodiversity: The Dasgupta Review*. London: HM Treasury; 2021.

58. New Zealand Government. *The Wellbeing Budget*. Wellington: New Zealand Government; 2019.

59. Davies SC. *Annual Report of the Chief Medical Officer 2018: Health 2040—Better Health Within Reach*. London: Department of Health and Social Care; 2018.

60. Heneghan C, Mahtani KR. Is it time to end general health checks? *BMJ Evidence Based Medicine* 2019; *25*: 115–16.

61. Krogsboll LT, Jorgensen KJ, Gotzsche PC. General health checks in adults for reducing morbidity and mortality from disease. *Cochrane Database of Systematic Reviews* 2019; *1*: CD009009.

62. Perry H, Sheehan E, Thilaganathan B, Khalil A. Home blood-pressure monitoring in a hypertensive pregnant population. *Ultrasound in Obstetrics and Gynecology* 2018; *51*: 524–30.

63. Winn AN, Ekwueme DU, Guy GP, Jr., Neumann PJ. Cost-utility analysis of cancer prevention, treatment, and control: A systematic review. *American Journal of Preventive Medicine* 2016; *50*: 241–8.

64. Valle I, Tramalloni D, Bragazzi NL. Cancer prevention: State of the art and future prospects. *Journal of Preventive Medicine and Hygiene* 2015; *56*: E21–7.

65. Greenberg D, Earle C, Fang CH, Eldar-Lissai A, Neumann PJ. When is cancer care cost-effective? A systematic overview of cost-utility analyses in oncology. *Journal of the National Cancer Institute* 2010; *102*: 82–8.

66. Vargas AJ, Schully SD, Villani J, Ganoza Caballero L, Murray DM. Assessment of prevention research measuring leading risk factors and causes of mortality and disability supported by the US National Institutes of Health. *JAMA Network Open* 2019; *2*: e1914718.

67. Kenkel DS. The demand for preventive medical care. *Applied Economics* 1994; *26*: 313–25.

68. Lange F. The role of education in complex health decisions: Evidence from cancer screening. *Journal of Health Economics* 2011; *30*: 43–54.

69. Carrieri V, Bilger M. Preventive care: Underused even when free. Is there something else at work? *Applied Economics* 2013; *45*: 239–53.

70. Fineberg HV. The paradox of disease prevention: Celebrated in principle, resisted in practice. *Journal of the American Medical Association* 2013; *310*: 85–90.

71. Horwitz JR, Kelly BD, DiNardo JE. Wellness incentives in the workplace: Cost savings through cost shifting to unhealthy workers. *Health Affairs (Millwood)* 2013; *32*: 468–76.

72. Horwitz JR, Kelly BD, DiNardo JE. Workplace wellness: The authors reply. *Health Affairs (Millwood)* 2013; *32*: 1510.

73. Owusu-Addo E, Renzaho AMN, Smith BJ. The impact of cash transfers on social determinants of health and health inequalities in sub-Saharan Africa: A systematic review. *Health Policy and Planning* 2018; *33*: 675–96.

74. Yasar Y. The health insurance market, labor unions, and utilization of cancer screening. *The Social Science Journal* 2009; *46*: 319–34.

75. Zeegers Paget D, Renshaw N, Droogers M. What role can civil society organizations have in European health policy? *European Journal of Public Health* 2017; *27*: 52–5.

76. Gostin LO, Monahan JT, Kaldor J, et al. The legal determinants of health: Harnessing the power of law for global health and sustainable development. *Lancet* 2019; *393*: 1857–910.

77. World Health Organization. *Health in All Policies: Helsinki Statement. Framework for Country Action.* Geneva: World Health Organization; 2014.

78. Dye C. Expanded health systems for sustainable development. *Science* 2018; *359*: 1337–9.

79. Nilsson M, Griggs D, Visbeck M. Map the interactions between Sustainable Development Goals. *Nature* 2016; *534*: 320–2.

80. Nilsson M, Chisholm E, Griggs D, et al. Mapping interactions between the sustainable development goals: Lessons learned and ways forward. *Sustainability Science* 2018; *13*: 1489–503.

81. Mock CN, Smith KR, Kobusingye O, et al. Injury prevention and environmental health: Key messages from disease control priorities. 3rd edn. In: Mock CN, Nugent R, Kobusingye O, Smith KR, eds. *Injury Prevention and Environmental Health.* Washington, DC: World Bank; 2017: Chapter 1.

82. Brown V, Diomedi BZ, Moodie M, Veerman JL, Carter R. A systematic review of economic analyses of active transport interventions that include physical activity benefits. *Transport Policy* 2016; *45*: 190–208.

83. United Nations Economic Commission for Europe (UNECE). *SDGs and the UN Transport Conventions.* Geneva: UNECE; 2016.

84. Watkins DA, Nugent R, Saxenian H, et al. Intersectoral policy priorities for health. In: Jamison DT, Gelband H, et al., eds. *Disease Control Priorities: Improving Health and Reducing Poverty.* Washington, DC: World Bank; 2017: Chapter 2.

85. Mohammadi NK, Sayyari A, Farshad A, et al. From MDGs to SDGs: New impetus to advance health in Iran. *Health Scope* 2019; *8*: e86420.

86. Greszczuk C. *Implementing Health in All Policies.* London: The Health Foundation; 2019.

4

Unlikely disasters

It's impossible that the improbable will never happen.

Emil Gumbel (*Statistics of Extremes*, 1958)

Predictions of an apocalypse are rarely effective as a call to arms. If the threat of disaster—an earthquake, a pandemic, or a nuclear accident—is unlikely or uncertain in time, place, and scale, then prevention may not, in fact, be judged better than cure.[1]

Looking to the future, the improbable is usually given low priority. Doubt dilutes deterrence, even in the face of a fearful hazard. Reflecting on disasters past, the consequences of inaction are frequently a source of painful regret. United States Secretary of Health and Human Services Michael Leavitt remarked in 2007 that: 'Everything we do before a pandemic will seem alarmist. Everything we do after a pandemic will seem inadequate.' Leavitt's comment speaks to fundamental principles that the current coronavirus pandemic is unlikely to change (Chapter 2). The challenge, however, is not to change the principles: rather, it is to exploit them more effectively in the cause of prevention.

When the sound of alarm bells falls on deaf ears, the response is commonly to shout more loudly[2] and issue further statements of what heads of government, financial institutions, and the United Nations (UN) 'must' do.[3] There is a better, more rational approach: instead of re-issuing the same stark warnings and blunt directives, it is more productive to appeal to reason: to understand why the threat of a pandemic or some other grave danger fails to elicit action—why prevention is, in effect, not thought to be better than cure.

The Great Health Dilemma. Christopher Dye, Oxford University Press. © Oxford University Press 2021. DOI: 10.1093/oso/9780198853824.003.0004

Reason and rhetoric

The appeal to reason comes in three parts. First and most obviously, adopt the best technical practices when investigating outbreaks and emergencies, including the means of data collection, analysis, and reporting.[4,5] Second, draw extra power by combining knowledge and skills from different disciplines—epidemiology, social sciences, research and development, diplomacy, logistics, and crisis management.[6] And third—the focus of this chapter—understand how choices and decisions are made in the face of unlikely disasters, based not only on the facts about hazards and risks, but also on the perceptions, values, and motives of all those who have a stake.[5]

COVID-19, a pandemic of a severe acute respiratory syndrome caused by the coronavirus SARS-CoV-2, has regenerated the argument that there is no trade-off between protecting health and protecting the economy. The leaders of the World Health Organization (WHO) and the International Monetary Fund contend that protecting public health and putting people back to work go hand-in-hand—rhetorically, to save lives is also to save livelihoods.[7]

'No trade-off' implies that the costs of intervening are less than the benefits (i.e. the averted costs of not intervening). How these costs and benefits are calculated, and how they are perceived, depends on the way health and wealth are valued, over what time period, and with respect to what part of the economy. As COVID-19 swept through New York in April 2020, Governor Andrew Cuomo declared that 'we're not going to put a dollar figure on human life'.[8] And yet, like it or not, values are placed on life all the time, implicitly and explicitly.

Faced with an emergency, the general goal is to maximize benefits in relation to costs, whether or not there are net savings. On the scale of national economies, countries with swifter and more forceful responses ('lockdown') to COVID-19, such as Austria, Germany, Japan, and the Republic of Korea, reported fewer deaths and smaller reductions in gross domestic product per capita.[9,10] Although expenditure on, and as a consequence of, COVID-19 control is not made explicit in such analyses, the implication is that early intervention has been a win–win: earlier lockdowns saved more lives at a lower cost to the economy. The short-term pain incurred was purportedly less than the longer-term pain averted.

During the COVID-19 lockdowns in March and April of 2020, the implicit value placed on a human life in both the United Kingdom and United States was high—by one estimate, around 10 times higher than the

Organisation for Economic Co-operation and Development's US$1.5–4.5 million 'value of a statistical life' (Box 2.1).[11] At that time, the UK lockdown policy appeared to be in step with public preferences for health over wealth. A separate analysis for the US, based on the impact of COVID-19 on economic productivity, also calculated that the benefits of control policies would, on these terms, probably exceed the costs.[12]

And yet the price of shutting down societies and economies to contain COVID-19 has been high in absolute terms—and very high when the lockdowns have been prolonged or repeated. On trade, shutting national borders stops the importation of infections but also interrupts the exchange of goods.[8] On education, closing schools protects children, teachers, and the rest of society from infection, but hinders learning and the social and psychological development of children, with longer-term effects on their skills and incomes. Keeping children out of school also jeopardizes the earnings of parents who must stay home to look after them. Poorer families are less resilient financially, amplifying inequalities.[13]

At the start of 2021, it looks unlikely that COVID-19 can be eradicated from the human population—SARS-CoV-2 infection will become endemic around the world, perhaps with local and temporary elimination (unlike SARS-CoV-1, which was eradicated from the human population after an outbreak in 2002). The challenge is to keep COVID-19 at low levels by means other than costly lockdowns of society. There are now better ways to prevent infection and illness, led by vaccination for all, backed by improved diagnostics for efficient testing (with isolation) and contact tracing (with quarantine) during outbreaks, and supported by improved curative treatments.

Against the backdrop of COVID-19, the rest of this chapter considers how best to prevent or manage any unlikely disaster—given the hazard, the risk, the options for containing it, and the associated costs.

Hazard: Real and perceived danger

The facts about a given hazard—the duration of illness, the level of pain and disability caused, the chance of dying, the months or years of life lost—can all be assessed by standard methods, which are widely used (Box 2.1).

But public health needs public participation, which depends, in turn, on public perception. A hazard often generates more concern, and is more likely to elicit a response, when the illness or injury has a fearful cause (sharks, snakes, and spiders), when the medical effects are gruesome (viral fevers that cause bleeding such as Ebola and Marburg virus diseases, Crimean-Congo haemorrhagic fever), when children are more likely to be affected than adults (pandemic H1N1 influenza), and when the hazard is new, changing, uncertain, or uncontrollable (emerging diseases including COVID-19; Chapter 2). Compared with familiar endemic infections— malaria, tuberculosis (Chapter 5), and diarrheal diseases (Chapter 7)— emerging epidemic diseases appear disproportionately threatening when judged against objective measures such as the number of people who become severely ill or die.

A heightened sense of threat is a stimulus for action but also requires the productive management of information produced by different means on different timescales. News of an emerging pathogen excites rapid but transient interest among the general public, although this influences government control policies. The timescale of the public response to COVID-19, rising and falling within a few weeks (Figure 4.1a), was similar to that for previous epidemics of Ebola, MERS (Middle East respiratory syndrome), SARS (caused by SARS-CoV-1) and pandemic influenza.[14,15] The mixed content of public debate is more and less positive for health: pronouncements by authoritative public bodies such as WHO are offset by messages promoting conspiracy theories, fear, stigma, and misinformation.[16]

The 'infodemic' of misinformation is a challenge to the methods proposed in this book. If perceptions influence choices, they have a place in the analysis of costs and benefits, but some opinions stretch beyond the standard methods of economic evaluation (Box 2.1). Among these subjective evaluations, the task is to decide which to include or exclude.

Scientific research is more uniformly positive for health, and driven by need, but produces information more slowly. The number of scientific papers on coronaviruses published annually increased after the SARS outbreak began in 2002, then subsided until the emergence of MERS in 2012, but never exceeded 1,000 publications per year. The COVID-19 pandemic dramatically changed the dynamics of coronavirus research: publications exploded early in 2020, and were averaging around 800 per week between May and September (Figure 4.1b). This is the supply of science that swiftly responded to the demand for new ways to control coronavirus diseases, specifically COVID-19.

A hazard has a public higher profile when formally classified as a major threat. A Public Health Emergency of International Concern (PHEIC) is a 'serious, sudden, unusual, or unexpected' cross-border risk to health. When

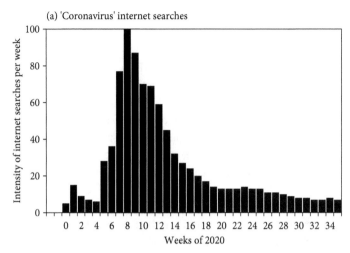

(a) 'Coronavirus' internet searches

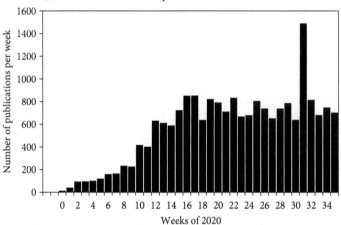

(b) Number of 'coronavirus' publications

Figure 4.1 Reponses to the new coronavirus, the cause of COVID-19, on different timescales. (a) Shorter: weekly intensity of worldwide internet searches for 'coronavirus', compared with the maximum (scaled to 100 in week 8). (b) Longer: weekly numbers of scientific papers on 'coronavirus' published worldwide.

Source: Data from National Center for Biotechnology Information. LitCovid. 2020. https://www.ncbi.nlm.nih.gov/research/coronavirus/docsum?text=coronavirus; Google Trends. Coronavirus. 2020. https://trends.google.com/trends/explore?q=%2Fm%2F01cpyy&geo=US

an epidemic is framed as a matter of national security, it will be managed on the same level as counter-terrorism.[15,17,18] The 2014–16 West African Ebola epidemic was a PHEIC and a security risk. On top of the public health response, US and UK military involvement drew vastly more resources than is typically available for epidemic control: US$5.9 billion was disbursed by 77 donors in 2014–15.[19] However, foreign assistance to combat Ebola subsided as the security threat beyond West Africa diminished. The bulk of 2014–15 donations (79%) was spent on the emergency response. Only 18% of funds (compared with 40% pledged) were targeted at longer-term recovery, including primary health care and preparedness for future outbreaks, and only 3% were reserved for research and development into future means of Ebola prevention and treatment.[19,20]

The security label carries another risk, if accompanied by secrecy at a time when accurate data are needed locally, immediately, and publicly for effective disease control. In this context, specialized biosecurity centres risk duplicating instead of reinforcing national public health infrastructures, including networks of health protection teams and diagnostic laboratories.[18]

Because a bigger threat is likely to stimulate a bigger response, there is a temptation towards hazard inflation. One example is antimicrobial or antibiotic resistance (AMR). There is no question that AMR is a threat to the health of people everywhere (Chapter 5).[21] However, an influential report published in 2016 concluded that, if AMR is not addressed, antibiotic resistant bacteria could claim 10 million lives each year by 2050.[22] This estimate is not justified either by the data or by the analysis used to produce it.[23] Nor it is plausible in view of the long-term decline in deaths from infections (fewer than 8 million in total in 2018). It remains to be seen whether the short-term benefits of exaggerating the AMR hazard—one of which was the UN's declaration on AMR in September 2016—prove detrimental to the longer-term credibility of the science, ultimately weakening rather than strengthening the case for action.

Risk: A problem shared

Almost all hazards can be managed if the cost is commensurate with the avoidable risk (Chapter 2). When all individuals in a population are at risk of a defined hazard, but only a small fraction will be affected by it, the general tactic is to pool the risk and share the cost. This is the basis of the insurance industry. Here we are most concerned with health insurance to preserve health rather than to remedy illness.

What follows are six ways, among others, of providing insurance against an emergency. They are all ways of encouraging investment in primary or secondary prevention, though none are exclusively preventive.

All the X in one basket

The first solution is to tackle emerging infections, not as separate, unpredictable events, but as a collective threat—that is, pool the risks of multiple hazards. Between 2011 and 2018, WHO tracked 1,483 epidemics in 72 countries, including Ebola, SARS and pandemic influenza (Figure 4.2).[24] Although human infectious disease outbreaks have been increasing over the past four decades,[25] the number of events recorded by WHO in 2011–18 was predictable within narrow bounds, averaging 185 (range 154–213) per year.

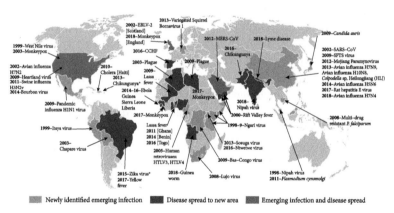

Figure 4.2 Global map of emerging infections 1997–2018. The number of infectious disease outbreaks worldwide every year is large and predictable, but the cause, timing, and magnitude of each outbreak is uncertain. A global overview opens the way to managing the combined hazard of multiple, low-risk, high-impact events.

Reproduced from Public Health England (PHE). (2019). Emerging infections: how and why they arise. London, UK: Public Health England. © Crown Copyright. Contains public sector information licensed under the Open Government Licence v3.0. https://www.nationalarchives.gov.uk/doc/open-government-licence/version/3/

To help prioritize research and development (R&D) investment among all these hazards, WHO has listed the world's top 10 emerging disease threats, which in August 2020 were COVID-19, Crimean-Congo haemorrhagic fever, Ebola and Marburg virus diseases, Lassa fever, MERS and SARS, Nipah and henipaviral diseases, Rift Valley fever, and Zika.[26]

Also on the list is anonymous 'Disease X' to make the point that the next emergency could be caused by an unknown pathogen from an unknown source with unknown consequences. Disease X could arise through multiple routes: viral or bacterial mutation; zoonotic pathogens that jump from animals to humans; or construction in a laboratory.

Ideally, we would stop epidemics, pandemics, and other disasters from happening at all, through primary prevention targeting these multiple threats. Over the decade 2009–19, the US Agency for International Development spent US$170 million on evaluating the 'feasibility of pre-emptively mitigating pandemic threats', via the Global Virome Project (GVP).[27] Even though a novel human pathogen is likely to be of animal origin (three-quarters are zoonotic) and most likely to be a virus,[28,29] the chance of identifying the next pathogen by screening the entire global virome is small.[30] The animal viruses that have the potential to infect people would have to be found among millions of undiscovered virus species. The search might be more fruitful if focused on especially risky pathogens, notably mammalian RNA viruses.[31,32] However, not even retrospective analyses of COVID-19 have identified the pathway of coronavirus SARS-CoV-2 from animals to humans. Viral emergence from animal reservoirs is still largely unpredictable and unpreventable.[33]

Here as elsewhere, there is an extra catch to primary prevention, besides the inefficiency of searching for prospective pathogens: the reward for effort is essentially invisible (Chapter 2). Projects such as GVP will certainly advance virology, but the main epidemiological measure of success is that nothing happens.

There are other more practical options, which include a mix of primary and secondary prevention: the early detection and control of pathogen spillovers from wild animals to domestic animals or humans; the regulation of trade in wildlife and bush meat; and the control of deforestation (where humans contact animal sources of infection).[34,35] Halting deforestation also preserves carbon stores and limits greenhouse gas emissions. The cost of this package of interventions (US$22–31 billion per year) was estimated, in one assessment, to be substantially smaller than the cost of future pandemics.[34] Whether this argument will lead to action depends on the willingness to pay for these interventions, their effectiveness in practice, and perceptions of the benefits, including how lives are valued in the present and in future.

If and when pathogens escape early interception, health services need to be prepared and protected. WHO's Technical Guidelines for Integrated Disease Surveillance and Response in the African Region (IDSR) explain how to respond rapidly to any disease outbreak,[36] and the West African Ebola epidemic (2014–16) showed how IDSR can work well if methodically implemented.[20,37,38] Between July and November 2014, 12 Ebola outbreaks in Liberia were investigated in a variant of IDSR, the Rapid Isolation and Treatment of Ebola (RITE) strategy. Active case finding and contact tracing were central to RITE, together with methods to protect those caring for the sick and burying the dead. In a comparison of the effects of six outbreaks that occurred before the introduction of RITE and six that occurred afterwards, the time between the first new case in remote areas and the notification of health authorities was reduced by nearly half, the proportion of patients isolated increased from 28% to 81%, survival improved from 13% to 50%, the case reproduction number fell below unity (the threshold for disease persistence), outbreaks became shorter (median duration declined from 53 to 25 days), and the number of generations of cases dropped from a median of four to two. These do not provide the strength of evidence afforded by a randomized controlled trial, but the findings are consistent with the larger body of evidence on Ebola interventions.

On a global scale, the Commission on a Global Health Risk Framework for the Future (2016) calculated that the loss to society from potential pandemics is more than US$60 billion each year, with a 10% chance that the loss could be more than twice that amount. To counter that loss, they proposed spending an extra US$4.5 billion per year in preparing for pandemics—or 65 cents per person.[15,39] A large part of that sum, US$3.4 billion, would be used to upgrade public health infrastructure and capabilities in low- and middle-income countries—an insurance policy covering a wide range of risks to health (cf. specialized biosecurity centres).[18] Another US$1 billion would fund research and development for epidemic diseases. The 65 cents per person looks like good value for money, but the costs and benefits are incurred by and accrue to different people. Given all the other worthy causes in the world, wealthy donors might also ask how they could better spend $4.5 billion per year, even if it amounts to just a few cents per person.

The notion of insuring against health emergencies has been explored in a diversity of schemes. Some ideas, such as Development Impact Bonds

(DIBs) and Social Impact Bonds (SIBs), have not yet become mainstream practice. DIBs and SIBs are three-way contracts in which private investors finance development and social programmes, an agency (often public sector) delivers the programme, and governments (SIBs) or donors (DIBs) eventually pay back investors. The payback is the principal plus a return, which is provided if, and only if, the programme succeeds in achieving its goals.[40,41]

Health interventions of proven effectiveness should be attractive to capital-rich investors. The prevention of African sleeping sickness, transmitted by tsetse flies, is a case in point.[42] *Trypanosoma brucei rhodesiense* is a pathogen of animals, including cattle, that occasionally spills over to humans, for whom it is almost always fatal. The mass treatment of cattle with trypanocidal drugs, followed by the application of insecticides to deter tsetse flies, gives a double benefit, preventing infection in valuable livestock and susceptible people (another example of 'treatment as prevention'; Chapter 5). The successful use of DIBs for sleeping sickness could open the way for other similar applications, such as vaccination to prevent rabies in domestic dogs and people. However, DIBs have not yet been used for the prevention of sleeping sickness, rabies, or any other infectious disease.

Some innovative insurance mechanisms have failed practical tests. The World Bank's Pandemic Emerging Finance Facility (PEF) has its origins in 'catastrophe bonds', putative instruments for insuring against disasters such as hurricanes.[43] The intention of PEF was to persuade insurance companies to take on some of the risk posed by catastrophic epidemics of Ebola, coronaviruses, influenza, and other infectious diseases. But PEF has hit two major snags.[44,45] One is that the trigger for payouts to affected countries is too slow—the money is provided only when an outbreak has satisfied a complex set of epidemiological criteria. A slow response to a rapidly expanding epidemic means that many people could become seriously ill or die before any funding is received. It is an ineffective method of prevention. The other is that interest payments have been unduly favourable to rich-country investors, leading to the charge that PEF bonds are overpriced handouts to speculators.[46] By July 2020, PEF had paid out roughly US$150 million to 48 countries affected by COVID-19. At around the same time, the World Bank announced that it would not issue any further bonds.

The World Bank disburses far more money through simpler mechanisms, such as those linking disbursement directly to programme results. Between 2012 and 2019, more than a hundred such operations had received around US$30 billion.[47] Many of the projects funded by this mechanism alleviate the collective risks of illness in a different way—for example, by strengthening health, water, and sanitation systems in low-income countries.

Inclusive risk

The argument for preventing a health hazard is more compelling when a large number of people are at risk, not just the marginalized few. In the US in 1981, cases of a rare lung infection, *Pneumocystis carinii pneumonia (PCP)*, were found in five young, previously healthy, gay men in Los Angeles. This was the first report of HIV/AIDS, which was initially known publicly as a 'gay disease' and medically as 'gay-related immune deficiency syndrome' (GRID).

HIV/AIDS was also known to be a disease of haemophiliacs as early as 1981. But in 1984, Ryan White, a haemophiliac teenager from Indiana, was excluded from school after becoming infected through contaminated blood. White's advocacy for AIDS research and awareness helped break the stigma of HIV/AIDS as a gay disease. In January 1983, HIV/AIDS was reported among female partners of infected men showing that the virus was heterosexually transmissible too. Throughout the 1980s, it became clear that HIV/AIDS was a threat to everyone, not only in the US but worldwide.

The Ryan White CARE Act (Comprehensive AIDS Resources Emergency Act) passed by Congress in 1990, the year of White's death, has since become the largest federally funded programme in the US for people living with HIV/AIDS. It was also a precursor to the creation of the United States Leadership Against Global HIV/AIDS, Tuberculosis, and Malaria Act of 2003, which in turn created the President's Emergency Plan for AIDS Relief (PEPFAR). PEPFAR is the largest commitment ever by any nation for an international health initiative dedicated to a single disease.

Technology platforms

The 2014–16 West African Ebola epidemic demonstrated the strengths and weaknesses of doing research during a health emergency. Building on prior research funded by the governments of Canada and the US, two safe and efficacious vaccines were developed as products of a global public–private collaboration including international health organizations, national governments and their public health agencies, field response and non-governmental organizations, universities, and pharmaceutical companies.[48,49]

In fact, better preparedness might have led to greater successes in the development of both vaccines and therapies for Ebola. In particular, trials of antiviral drugs and immune therapies (convalescent plasma) yielded no conclusive results on efficacy, and progress in developing Ebola therapies since then has been slow.[50,51] These sub-optimal results leave open the question of how discovery, development, and deployment can be accelerated, in view of repeated Ebola outbreaks, notably in the Democratic Republic of Congo in 2018–21.

The decision to invest in making new health technologies—diagnostics, drugs, machines, reagents, vaccines—depends on the chance of developing an effective product and the size of the potential market, among other factors. From the perspective of pharmaceutical companies, the development of vaccines (preventive) is generally less rewarding than drugs (curative), as reflected in the vastly different size of their global markets. Drugs are a trillion dollar market annually whereas vaccines bring revenues of around US$50 billion.[52] The simplest explanation for the difference is that an effective vaccine is given just once to each person at risk whereas drugs can be prescribed repeatedly.

That difference is exacerbated by another characteristic of prevention and cure. In any population exposed to a hazard, the risk is generally distributed unevenly—a few people are at high risk while many are at low risk.[53] The advantage of a curative drug is that the distribution of risk can be observed directly, as the outcome of exposure—a drug can be given to anyone who becomes sick. A preventive vaccine is at a comparative disadvantage if a manufacturer must decide whether to make a low-cost, high-volume product that can be sold to everyone, even people at low risk, or a high-cost, low-volume product targeting those at high risk. Faced with that trade-off, a vaccine is expected to generate less revenue than a drug.[54]

In principle, investment in vaccine development should be more appealing when co-funded (pooled risk), when a target product has multiple uses (applicable whatever Disease X turns out to be), and when it can be rapidly deployed (a readily adaptable product). Considering all these factors, the Coalition for Epidemic Preparedness Innovations (CEPI) was set up in 2017 to accelerate vaccine discovery, development, and deployment—a partnership between public, private, philanthropic, and civil society organizations.[55] Guided by WHO's list of top 10 targets for R&D (above),[56] shared investment aims to develop vaccines against the coronavirus diseases MERS, SARS, and COVID-19, plus Chikungunya, Ebola, Lassa, Nipah and Rift Valley fevers. CEPI puts the average minimum cost of developing at least one vaccine to phase 2a (producing initial data on short-term safety and efficacy) for each pathogen at $2.8–3.7 billion.

CEPI's operational model makes use of platform technologies. These rapid response platforms use a generic module based, for example, on a viral vector, or synthetic DNA or RNA, to deliver a gene that encodes an agent that induces protective immunity (Figure 4.3).[56,57] The platform is a template—one process that can be used, with minor alterations, to make different vaccines using a common technology.[58] The platform should enable manufacturers to develop new vaccines for specific pathogens more

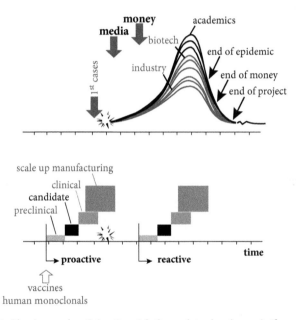

Figure 4.3 Sharing and anticipating risk through technology platforms. Top: the usual reactive steps in vaccine development and delivery, lagging behind the emergence of a single novel pathogen. Bottom: the earlier timing of a proactive approach to create generic platform technologies that are precursors for vaccines to prevent infection with a range of different pathogens ('Disease X').

Adapted with permission from Bloom, D.E., Black, S., Rappuoli, R. (2017). Emerging infectious diseases: A proactive approach. Proceedings of the National Academy of Sciences USA, 114: 4055–9.

quickly, to cut the cost of building manufacturing facilities, and perhaps to streamline regulatory processes. Conventional (e.g. inactivated and live viruses) and novel platforms (e.g. DNA and RNA) are now being used to develop vaccines against COVID-19, including universal vaccines with the potential to protect against all SARS-CoV-2 variants, and even pan-virus vaccines.[59,60]

COVAX, led by WHO, CEPI, and GAVI, the Vaccine Alliance is an international mechanism for sharing the costs, risks, and benefits of COVID-19 multiple initiatives for vaccine development. COVAX promises fair and equitable access for countries worldwide, especially low- and middle-income countries. And yet some countries chose to take a high stakes gamble: the European Union, UK, and US ordered millions of doses of unproven vaccine candidates. For the UK and US, this appears to have paid off: both countries achieved relatively high vaccination coverage by the end of February 2021.

Health regulations

Originating in Europe's nineteenth-century defence against cholera, the International Health Regulations (IHR 2005) is the only treaty governed by international law that is designed 'to prevent, protect against, control and provide a public health response to the international spread of disease'. Unlike the historical antecedents, the IHR 2005 is not limited to specific diseases (cholera, plague, yellow fever) but applies to new and ever-changing public health risks, including air pollution and nuclear accidents.[61] Under the IHR 2005, WHO has the power to declare a PHEIC, and has done so for the H1N1 'swine flu' pandemic in 2009, polio in 2014, Ebola in 2014 and 2018, Zika in 2015, and COVID-19 in 2020.

The signatories to the IHR 2005, the States Parties, are bound to notify to WHO all emergencies that pose an international threat, to permit verification, and to inform other States of the risks they face. The benefits are clear: by sharing information, the governments of affected countries can also share the cost of confronting a new hazard, receive technical assistance and logistical support, and gain access to new technologies.[62] No country can single-handedly develop diagnostics, drugs, or vaccines for Ebola, Zika, or COVID-19.

But disclosure carries costs as well as benefits. Governments may fear that external verification jeopardizes security or sovereignty, even if it comes with financial or technical support. They may be concerned that reporting an outbreak will lead to restrictions on the movement of people and goods between countries, with benefits for health but costs to the economy. Although the IHR 2005 stipulates that there should be no 'unnecessary interference with international traffic and trade', at least 30 countries did impose such restrictions on travellers from West Africa during the 2014–16 Ebola outbreak.[63] These regulations, restated during the epidemic by WHO, were ignored at the convenience of IHR signatories, and with impunity. One analysis of eight major disease events that occurred between 2013 and 2018 found 210 instances of governments implementing health measures that contravened the IHR 2005. The most frequent breech was to deny entry to international travellers.[64] During the COVID-19 pandemic, almost all countries have decided, with good reason, that restrictions on international travel are necessary to prevent the importation of infections, and have therefore restricted visas, closed borders, and imposed quarantine measures.[65]

Given the trade-offs between health, economy, sovereignty, and security, and the difficulties of enforcement, it is no surprise that compliance with the IHR 2005 has been poor, compromising the treaty as a mechanism for sharing costs and risks. A 2015 review found that 78 out of 196 countries failed to report on the IHR 2005 at all, and those that did report achieved low scores (between 55% and 87%) on core capacities. There were reporting gaps on antimicrobial resistance, biosafety and biosecurity, preparedness, emergency response operations, medical countermeasures and personnel deployment, and chemical events and radiation emergencies.[66,67]

These observations, reinforced by events during the COVID-19 pandemic, have reignited debate about how to make the IHR 2005 more effective. The suggestions include ways to clarify the criteria for declaring a PHEIC, eliminate legal ambiguities, embrace human rights, resolve disputes, and allow for the economics of travel and tourism as much as trade.[68,69] On the matter of resolving disputes, lessons can be drawn from the advances made in sharing intellectual and material property, as follows.

Intellectual and material property

Within the broad framework of the IHR 2005 lies the question of how to share information and materials to the benefit of individual owners of the data and the whole research community. These assets are often seen as public goods that should be made freely available, especially in an emergency. But intellectual and material property have commercial, political, and professional value. The governments of affected countries are concerned that biological data and materials will be used to produce treatments they cannot afford; scientists sharing data worry about losing credit for a discovery; and biotechnology companies want a stake in developing or manufacturing new diagnostics, drugs, and vaccines.[70]

In 2006, following a dispute over commercial vaccine development by a foreign company, Indonesia agreed to share samples of influenza A virus (H5N1, 'bird flu') on the condition that WHO and other countries guarantee access to vaccines derived from virus samples it provided.[71] This specific issue, framed as a matter of property and sovereignty in international law, eventually led to a general solution—the Pandemic Influenza Preparedness (PIP) Framework (2011). PIP is a charter for sharing H5N1 and other influenza viruses with human pandemic potential, and for providing access to vaccines. Several open access databases operate alongside PIP: one of these, the Global Initiative on Sharing Avian Influenza Data (GISAID), has become a primary source of genomic data, now including information on all influenza viruses and COVID-19.[72,73] GISAID has successfully attracted support by giving credit to those who contribute data and by ensuring that they benefit from the research. The PIP framework and other data platforms reflect the major advances that have been made since 2006 in sharing information and materials through negotiation for mutual benefit.[70,74]

Division of labour

While the slow and initially uncoordinated response to Ebola in West Africa during 2014 drew much criticism,[75,76] the creation of an overarching United Nations Mission for the Emergency Ebola Response (UNMEER) in September 2014 provided a coordinated mechanism for tackling the epidemic.

The purpose of UNMEER was to combine the powers of UN agencies with different but complementary kinds of expertise (Figure 4.4). WHO provided technical expertise (training of health workers, oversight of clinical care, case finding, contact tracing, and laboratory services), the World Food Programme covered logistics (e.g. building Ebola treatment units), the International Federation of the Red Cross managed burials, and the

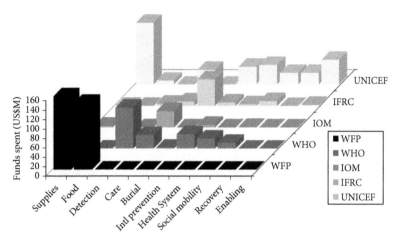

Figure 4.4 Division of labour. Coordinating the United Nations Mission for the Emergency Ebola Response (UNMEER) in West Africa by allocating international organizations according to their different but complementary types of expertise on supplies; food provision; case detection and care; burial; international aspects of prevention; health systems support; social mobilization; and epidemic recovery, and by enabling functions such as logistical support. World Food Programme (WFP); World Health Organization (WHO); Institute of Migration (IOM); International Federation of the Red Cross (IFRC); United Nations Children's Fund (UNICEF).

Source: Data from Office of the United Nations Special Envoy on Ebola. Resources for Results V. New York: Office of the United Nations Special Envoy on Ebola, 2016; WHO Ebola Response Team. After Ebola in West Africa: unpredictable risks, preventable epidemics *New England Journal of Medicine* 2016; 375: 587–96.

United Nations Children's Fund (UNICEF) coordinated social mobilization and health services. A high-profile launch of UNMEER at the UN Security Council and UN General Assembly in 2014 galvanized political support and helped to generate a funding stream. UNMEER received US$5.9 billion in donations, compared with the meagre US$155 million that had been provided up to September 2014.[77]

The establishment of a new organization mid-epidemic was not entirely smooth (cf. the creation of the UK National Institute for Health Protection during COVID-19; Chapter 3). The mission initially failed, for instance, to adjust for differences in organizational culture, especially between the UN's peacekeeping, humanitarian, and medical services. Nevertheless, the Ebola experience influenced the later restructuring of the WHO Health

Emergencies Programme and provided lessons for coordination among international agencies in future.

Summary

If the threat of disaster—an earthquake, a pandemic, or a nuclear accident—is unlikely or uncertain in time, place, and scale, then prevention may not be seen as better than cure. A potential health emergency becomes more manageable when the cost is commensurate with the hazard and the risk. Tactics to satisfy that criterion are familiar to the insurance industry: spotlight preventable hazards, pool the risks, and share the costs. A hazard—such as COVID-19, Ebola, or Zika virus—is perceived to be more dangerous, and more likely to stimulate action, when classified as a public health emergency or a threat to national security. Among the methods for pooling risks and sharing costs are: early detection and response systems for multiple pathogens; platform technologies for the development of new diagnostics and vaccines; collaborations through the IHR 2005; and shared genomic databases for bacteria and viruses.

References

1. Heymann DL, Dar OA. Prevention is better than cure for emerging infectious diseases. *BMJ* 2014; *348*: g1499.
2. Garrett L. The world knows an apocalyptic pandemic is coming but nobody is interested in doing anything about it. *Foreign Policy* 2019; 20 September.
3. Global Preparedness Monitoring Board. *A World in Disorder. Global Preparedness Monitoring Board Annual Report 2020*. Geneva: World Health Organization; 2020.
4. Polonsky JA, Baidjoe A, Kamvar ZN, et al. Outbreak analytics: A developing data science for informing the response to emerging pathogens. *Philosophical Transactions of the Royal Society B* 2019; *374*: 20180276.
5. Shearer FM, Moss R, McVernon J, Ross JV, McCaw JM. Infectious disease pandemic planning and response: Incorporating decision analysis. *PLoS Medicine* 2020; *17*: e1003018.
6. Bedford J, Farrar J, Ihekweazu C, Kang G, Koopmans M, Nkengasong J. A new twenty-first century science for effective epidemic response. *Nature* 2019; *575*: 130–6.
7. Georgieva K, Ghebreyesus TA. Some say there is a trade-off: Save lives or save jobs—this is a false dilemma. The Telegraph. 3 April 2020.

8. The Economist.Covid-19 presents stark choices between life, death and the economy. The Economist. 2 April 2020.
9. Hasell J. Which countries have protected both health and the economy in the pandemic? 2020. https://ourworldindata.org/covid-health-economy (accessed 7 January 2021).
10. Dye C, Cheng RCH, Dagpunar JS, Williams BG. The scale and dynamics of COVID-19 epidemics across Europe. Royal Society Open Science 2021; 7: 201726.
11. Hargreaves Heap SP, Koop C, Matakos K, Unan A, Weber N. Valuating health vs wealth: The effect of information and how this matters for COVID-19 policy-making. 2020. https://voxeu.org/article/health-vs-wealth-trade-and-covid-19-policymaking (accessed 7 January 2021).
12. Broughel J, Kotrous M. *The Benefits of Coronavirus Suppression: A Cost-Benefit Analysis of the Response to the First Wave of COVID-19*. Arlington, VA: Mercatus Center at George Mason University; 2020.
13. Edmunds WJ. Finding a path to reopen schools during the COVID-19 pandemic. *Lancet Child and Adolescent Health* 2020; published online 8 August.
14. Bento AI, Nguyen T, Wing C, Lozano-Rojas F, Ahn YY, Simon K. Evidence from internet search data shows information-seeking responses to news of local COVID-19 cases. *Proceedings of the National Academy of Sciences USA* 2020; *117*: 11220–2.
15. Sands P, Mundaca-Shah C, Dzau VJ. The neglected dimension of global security: A framework for countering infectious-disease crises. *New England Journal of Medicine* 2016; *374*: 1281–7.
16. Szmuda T, Ali S, Hetzger TV, Rosvall P, Sloniewski P. Are online searches for the novel coronavirus (COVID-19) related to media or epidemiology? A cross-sectional study. *International Journal of Infectious Diseases* 2020; *97*: 386–90.
17. Heymann DL, Chen L, Takemi K, et al. Global health security: The wider lessons from the west African Ebola virus disease epidemic. *Lancet* 2015; *385*: 1884–901.
18. Vize R. England's new covid-19 monitoring outfit: The Joint Biosecurity Centre. *BMJ* 2020; *370*: m2604.
19. Office of the United Nations Special Envoy on Ebola. *Resources for Results V*. New York: Office of the United Nations Special Envoy on Ebola; 2016.
20. WHO Ebola Response Team. After Ebola in West Africa: Unpredictable risks, preventable epidemics. *New England Journal of Medicine* 2016; *375*: 587–96.
21. World Health Organization. Antimicrobial resistance. 2020. https://www.who.int/health-topics/antimicrobial-resistance (accessed 7 January 2021).
22. O'Neill J. *Tackling Drug-Resistant Infections Globally: Final Report and Recommendations*. London: HM Government; 2016.
23. de Kraker ME, Stewardson AJ, Harbarth S. Will 10 million people die a year due to antimicrobial resistance by 2050? *PLoS Medicine* 2016; *13*: e1002184.
24. Global Preparedness Monitoring Board. *A World at Risk: Annual Report on Global Preparedness for Health Emergencies*. Geneva: World Health Organization; 2019.
25. Smith KF, Goldberg M, Rosenthal S, et al. Global rise in human infectious disease outbreaks. *Journal of the Royal Society Interface* 2014; *11*: 20140950.

26. World Health Organization. Prioritizing diseases for research and development in emergency contexts. https://www.who.int/activities/prioritizing-diseases-for-research-and-development-in-emergency-contexts (accessed 7 January 2021).

27. Carroll D, Daszak P, Wolfe ND, et al. The Global Virome Project. *Science 2018*; *359*: 872–4.

28. Woolhouse ME, Gowtage-Sequeria S. Host range and emerging and reemerging pathogens. *Emerging Infectious Diseases* 2005; *11*: 1842–7.

29. Woolhouse M, Scott F, Hudson Z, Howey R, Chase-Topping M. Human viruses: Discovery and emergence. *Philosophical Transactions of the Royal Society B* 2012; *367*: 2864–71.

30. Holmes EC, Rambaut A, Andersen KG. Pandemics: Spend on surveillance, not prediction. *Nature* 2018; *558*: 180–2.

31. Woolhouse MEJ, Adair K. The diversity of human RNA viruses. *Future Virology* 2013; *8*: 159–71.

32. Babayan SA, Orton RJ, Streicker DG. Predicting reservoir hosts and arthropod vectors from evolutionary signatures in RNA virus genomes. *Science* 2018; *362*: 577–80.

33. Streicker DG, Gilbert AT. Contextualizing bats as viral reservoirs. *Science* 2020; *370*: 172–3.

34. Dobson AP, Pimm SL, Hannah L, et al. Ecology and economics for pandemic prevention. *Science* 2020; *369*: 379–81.

35. Gibb R, Redding DW, Chin KQ, et al. Zoonotic host diversity increases in human-dominated ecosystems. *Nature* 2020; *584*: 398–402.

36. World Health Organization Regional Office for Africa and Centers for Disease Control and Prevention USA. *Technical Guidelines for Integrated Disease Surveillance and Response in the African Region*, 3rd edition. Brazzaville and Atlanta: World Health Organization Regional Office for Africa and Centers for Disease Control and Prevention USA; 2010.

37. Lindblade KA, Kateh F, Nagbe TK, et al. Decreased Ebola transmission after rapid response to outbreaks in remote areas, Liberia, 2014. *Emerging infectious diseases* 2015; *21*: 1800–7.

38. Kateh F, Nagbe T, Kieta A, et al. Rapid response to Ebola outbreaks in remote areas—Liberia, July–November 2014. *MMWR Morbidity and Mortality Weekly Report* 2015; *64*: 188–92.

39. Commission on a Global Health Risk Framework for the Future. *The Neglected Dimension of Global Security: A Framework to Counter Infectious Disease Crises.* Washington, DC: Commission on a Global Health Risk Framework for the Future; 2016.

40. Center for Global Development. Investing in social outcomes: Development Impact Bonds. 2020. https://www.cgdev.org/page/investing-social-outcomes-development-impact-bonds-0 (accessed 7 January 2021).

41. Center for Global Development. *Development Impact Bond Working Group Report: Consultation Draft.* Washington, DC: Center for Global Development; 2013.

42. Welburn SC, Bardosh KL, Coleman PG. Novel financing model for neglected tropical diseases: Development impact bonds applied to sleeping sickness and rabies control. *PLoS Neglected Tropical Diseases* 2016; *10*: e0005000.

43. Lewis M. In nature's casino. New York Times. 26 August 2007.

44. Jonas O. Pandemic bonds: Designed to fail in Ebola. *Nature* 2019; *572*: 285.

45. Brim B, Wenham C. Pandemic emergency financing facility: struggling to deliver on its innovative promise. *BMJ* 2019; *367*: l5719.

46. Dizard J. Coronavirus strikes World Bank's 2017 catastrophe bonds. Financial Times. 6 February 2020.

47. World Bank. Program-for-Results financing (PforR). 2020. https://www.worldbank.org/en/programs/program-for-results-financing (accessed 7 January 2021).

48. Kadlec R. *Making History: The World's First FDA-Approved Ebola Vaccine*. Washington, DC: US Department of Health and Human Services, Office of the Assistant Secretary for Preparedness and Response; 2019.

49. Wolf J, Bruno S, Eichberg M, et al. Applying lessons from the Ebola vaccine experience for SARS-CoV-2 and other epidemic pathogens. *NPJ Vaccines* 2020; *5*: 51.

50. Iversen PL, Kane CD, Zeng X, et al. Recent successes in therapeutics for Ebola virus disease: No time for complacency. *Lancet Infectious Diseases* 2020; *20*: e231–e7.

51. National Academies of Sciences, Engineering and Medicine. *Integrating Clinical Research into Epidemic Response: The Ebola Experience*. Washington, DC: National Academies Press; 2017.

52. Xue QC, Ouellette LL. Innovation policy and the market for vaccines. *Journal of Law and the Biosciences* 2020; *7*: lsaa026.

53. Woolhouse ME, Dye C, Etard JF, et al. Heterogeneities in the transmission of infectious agents: Implications for the design of control programs. *Proceedings of the National Academy of Sciences USA* 1997; *94*: 338–42.

54. Kremer M, Snyder CM. Preventives versus treatments. *The Quarterly Journal of Economics* 2015; *130*: 1167–239.

55. Bloom DE, Black S, Rappuoli R. Emerging infectious diseases: A proactive approach. *Proceedings of the National Academy of Sciences USA* 2017; *114*: 4055–9.

56. The Coalition for Epidemic Preparedness Innovations (CEPI). New vaccines for a safer world. 2020. https://cepi.net (accessed 7 January 2021).

57. World Health Organization. *An R&D Blueprint for Action to Prevent Epidemics*. Geneva: World Health Organization; 2016.

58. Adalja AA, Watson M, Cicero A, Inglesby T. *Vaccine Platforms: State of the Field and Looming Challenges*. Baltimore: Johns Hopkins University; 2019.

59. van Riel D, de Wit E. Next-generation vaccine platforms for COVID-19. *Nature Materials* 2020; *19*: 810–2.

60. Krammer, F. SARS-CoV-2 vaccines in development. *Nature* 2020; *586*: 516–27.

61. World Health Organization. *International Health Regulations (2005)*. 3rd edn. Geneva: World Health Organization; 2005.

62. World Health Organization. *Frequently asked Questions about the International Health Regulations (2005)*. Geneva: World Health Organization; 2009.
63. Pattani R. Unsanctioned travel restrictions related to Ebola unravel the global social contract. *CMAJ* 2015; *187*: 166–7.
64. Kamradt-Scott A, Dolea C, Ponce C, et al. WHO tracking mechanism for IHR additional health measures. *Lancet* 2018; *392*: 2250–1.
65. Lee K, Worsnop CZ, Grepin KA, Kamradt-Scott A. Global coordination on cross-border travel and trade measures crucial to COVID-19 response. *Lancet* 2020; *395*: 1593–5.
66. Suthar AB, Allen LG, Cifuentes S, Dye C, Nagata JM. Lessons learnt from implementation of the International Health Regulations: A systematic review. *Bulletin of the World Health Organization* 2018; *96*: 110–21.
67. Talisuna A, Yahaya AA, Rajatonirina SC, et al. Joint external evaluation of the International Health Regulation (2005) capacities: Current status and lessons learnt in the WHO African region. *BMJ Global Health* 2019; *4*: e001312.
68. Taylor AL, Habibi R, Burci GL, et al. Solidarity in the wake of COVID-19: Reimagining the International Health Regulations. *Lancet* 2020; *396*: 82–3.
69. Meier BM, Huffstetler HE, Habibi R. Human rights must be central to the International Health Regulations. *Health and Human Rights Journal* 2020; 26 August.
70. Goldacre B, Harrison S, Mahtani KR, Heneghan C. *Background Briefing for WHO Consultation on Data and Results Sharing during Public Health Emergencies*. Oxford: Centre for Evidence-Based Medicine, University of Oxford; 2015.
71. Fidler DP. Influenza virus samples, international law, and global health diplomacy. *Emerging Infectious Diseases* 2008; *14*: 88–94.
72. GISAID. 2020. https://www.gisaid.org (accessed 7 January 2021).
73. World Health Organization. *Pandemic Influenza Preparedness Framework for the Sharing of Influenza Viruses and Access to Vaccines and Other Benefits*. Geneva: World Health Organization; 2011.
74. Eccleston-Turner M, Phelan A, Katz R. Preparing for the next pandemic—The WHO's global influenza strategy. *New England Journal of Medicine* 2019; *381*: 2192–4.
75. *Ebola Interim Assessment Panel. Report of the Ebola Interim Assessment Panel*. Geneva: World Health Organization; 2015.
76. Maurice J. Expert panel slams WHO's poor showing against Ebola. *Lancet* 2015; *386*: e1.
77. Lupel A, Snyder M. *The Mission to Stop Ebola: Lessons for UN Crisis Response*. New York: International Peace Institute; 2017.

5
Normal ways to die

Tuberculosis is killing someone every 22 seconds.

The TB Alliance (2019)[1]

A tuberculosis death every 22 seconds adds up to 1.4 million lives lost annually. That makes *Mycobacterium tuberculosis* the biggest cause of death from a single infectious agent worldwide. And yet TB, like other everyday endemic diseases, is rarely seen as a health emergency. Tackling the pandemic of TB and other neglected diseases begins, not by insisting that millions of deaths constitute a crisis, but by understanding why they are acceptably normal.

Familiarity breeds neglect

Despite the millions of deaths each year, TB is generally perceived to be an unexceptional threat to health. From a public standpoint, the risk of illness and death from TB is low—as a global average, about 2 in 10,000 people die from TB each year. And although TB ranked thirteenth among causes of death in 2017, the disease accounts for a small part of the burden of illness that falls on communities and their health services—about 2 in 10,000 illnesses and 2 in 100 deaths in the global population each year.[2]

The International Health Regulations (IHR 2005) can, in principle, be used to help contain the worldwide spread of TB.[3] But unlike Ebola, Zika and COVID-19, it is improbable that TB will ever be classified as a Public Health Emergency of International Concern (PHEIC) under the IHR 2005 (Chapter 4). TB is present in most months of the year in most countries in the world; if the 1.4 million deaths that occur annually happened in a single month at an unpredictable location, the response would surely be far greater, and not simply because health services would be overwhelmed.

The Great Health Dilemma. Christopher Dye, Oxford University Press. © Oxford University Press 2021.
DOI: 10.1093/oso/9780198853824.003.0005

TB has another problem of perception: as for other endemic diseases, and unlike epidemic diseases, normal is not notable. A comparison with Ebola makes the point (Chapter 4). During the West African Ebola crisis of 2014–16—an unpredictable outbreak of a dreaded disease—the costs of managing the epidemic in Guinea, Liberia, and Sierra Leone, and the full economic costs of the epidemic, were about the same as for TB worldwide (Table 5.1). The estimated number of TB deaths in the three West African countries was of roughly the same magnitude as those for Ebola (both around 10,000), but the global death toll from TB was more than 100 times greater.

As a hazard to individuals, TB is intrinsically less fearful than some other threats to health and life. Advocates of TB control are fond of counting the number of lives lost from TB in units of crashed jumbo jets. But that statistic misses a key point: a plane crash incites a far greater level of fear than TB, in part because airline passengers have no control over their fate.

Table 5.1 Estimated numbers of deaths from Ebola and tuberculosis, with expenditures and economic costs counted over a 12-month period in 2014 and 2015

	Ebola (W. Africa 2014–15)	Tuberculosis (Global 2014)
Expenditure (US$ bn)	5.9	6.8
Economic cost (US$ bn)	53	41
Deaths	11,310 —	9,700 (W. Africa) 1.33 million (Global)

Notes:

1. Ebola deaths are as reported during the whole of the West African epidemic, mostly in Guinea, Liberia and Sierra Leone. Ebola funding is the total disbursed by donors, September 2014 to October 2015 (World Health Organization Ebola Response Team. After Ebola in West Africa: Unpredictable risks, preventable epidemics. New England Journal of Medicine 2016; 375: 587–96).

2. The economic cost of the Ebola epidemic was estimated by Huber et al. (Huber C, Finelli L, Stevens W. The economic and social burden of the 2014 Ebola outbreak in West Africa. Journal of Infectious Diseases 2018; 218[suppl. 5]: S698–S704).

3. Tuberculosis (TB) deaths exclude those among HIV-infected people, as estimated by World Health Organization (WHO). TB funding is for drug-sensitive cases in the low- and middle-income countries that reported 97% of all cases globally in 2018 (WHO. Global Tuberculosis Report 2019. Geneva: WHO; 2019).

4. TB economic costs are the annual average for the period 2000–15 (Global TB Caucus. The Price of a Pandemic 2017. London: Global TB Caucus; 2017).

There is little tolerable margin for error on aircraft safety. News of every accident is broadcast worldwide. The huge investment in crash prevention, to meet internationally agreed safety standards, makes commercial flying almost risk-free (in 2019, there was one accident with fatalities per 2 million flights). In contrast, TB is a life-threatening but indolent and curable disease, and mainly a disease of adults (less emotively than children; Chapter 2).

Forgotten, but not gone

The chronic invisibility of endemic, unchanging illness and death—caused by TB among many other conditions—is an enduring challenge to public health (Chapters 2 and 6). One of the most successful responses in the past decade has been the joint branding of a group of about 20 (classifications differ and change) transmissible pathogens as 'neglected tropical diseases' (NTDs), including dengue, leishmaniasis, onchocerciasis (river blindness), schistosomiasis (bilharzia), and intestinal helminths (roundworm, hookworm, and others).[4] Amalgamating the risks, NTDs are presented as one big cause of disease that is less easily overlooked, rather than many small diseases each of which can be ignored (Chapter 4). TB is not formally a NTD and is not quite so neglected, having been recognized as one of the big three unconquered infectious diseases, along with HIV/AIDS and malaria.

Joining that triumvirate has brought some success but TB remains the poor relation of the other two, especially HIV/AIDS, both with regard to domestic funding (US$11 billion for TB versus US$20 billion for HIV/AIDS in low- and middle-income countries in 2017) and international donor assistance (US$1.7 billion for TB versus US$9.5 billion for HIV/AIDS in 2019).[5,6] This distribution is mirrored in allocations made by the Global Fund, the principal financing agency for the big three, which has split its US$12.7 billion 2020–22 budget as 18% for TB and 50% for HIV/AIDS.[7]

TB control has relied primarily on treatment with combinations of drugs (principally isoniazid and rifampicin) that patients must take for long periods without interruption, usually six months or more.[8] The term 'treatment as prevention' was first used for antiretroviral therapy (ART) for HIV/AIDS, but that dual purpose—curing illness and stopping the transmission of infection to others—applies to any communicable disease where illness coincides with or precedes infectiousness, including TB. In effect, this is secondary prevention (averting severe illness and death) and primary prevention combined (stopping the spread of infection; Box 2.2).

Combination chemotherapy for TB is treatment as prevention: the drug combinations kill drug-sensitive bacteria quickly, stopping transmission and greatly reducing the risk of death. But the decline in TB incidence is slow (rarely more than 10% per year) because most populations carry a large reservoir of latent infection (a quarter of the global population is infected).[9] Furthermore, drug treatment programmes most effectively interrupt transmission when patients can be detected early in the course of illness but, given the slow onset of disease, early diagnosis has been hard to achieve in many settings.[8,10]

Just as TB control has centred on drug treatment, so too has investment in research and development (R&D). In 2018, nearly a billion dollars (US$906 million) was spent on TB R&D: 37% of that total was allocated to drug discovery, including curative and prophylactic drugs.[11] In line with industry priorities in general (Chapter 4), less was spent on vaccine research, only 12% in 2018, even though a replacement for the century-old BCG (Bacille Calmette-Guérin) vaccine is much needed. Operational research (OR)—better ways to use existing tools—is also perennially underfunded, attracting only 13% of R&D funds in 2018. The financing challenge for OR starts with a lack of ambition: with reference to the *Global Plan to End TB*,[5] OR secured all the money asked for in 2018—about US$300 million—whereas drugs and vaccines received only 22% and 24%, respectively, of far larger budgets.[11]

The comparatively low investment in TB research, coupled with the practical difficulties of patient diagnosis and treatment, helps to explain why more people died of TB than HIV/AIDS in 2017 (1.2 million versus 0.95 million), and why TB deaths are declining more slowly than HIV/AIDS deaths (4% versus 9% per year, 2008–17; Figure 5.1a). They also help to explain why the rate of decline of TB, whether measured in terms of disease or death, is falling much too slowly to meet global control targets by 2030 (Figure 5.1b).[10,12] To compound the difficulties, COVID-19 disrupted routine TB services worldwide during 2020.[12]

The challenge of TB control, therefore, is to encourage investment in combating a persistent but low-risk, low-value hazard so as to accelerate the decline in illness and death. This chapter takes up that challenge, first by considering the various options for control. As in all other settings, the case for prevention versus treatment rests on the comparison of costs and benefits.

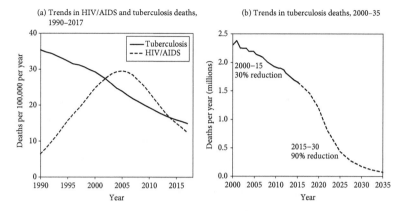

Figure 5.1 The challenge of tuberculosis (TB) prevention and treatment. (a) Global trends in deaths (per 100,000 population per year) from HIV/AIDS and TB. (b) Downward trends in the annual number of TB deaths (millions) observed over the period from 2000 to 2015, and projected 2015–30 in order to meet global targets for TB control.

Source: Data from World Health Organization. (2019). Global tuberculosis report 2019. Geneva, Switzerland: World Health Organization.

Prevention and cure

Table 5.1 summarizes the pros and cons of methods for TB control, along a spectrum from prevention to cure. For illustration, assume that drug treatment of active disease halves the basic case reproduction number, R_0, from 2 to 1 (R_0 is the number of secondary cases produced one primary case introduced to an uninfected population; when $R_0 \leq 1$, the disease can no longer persist).[8,13] This is equivalent to vaccination with an effectiveness of 50% (e.g. 80% of people vaccinated with 63% immunization efficacy in preventing infectious TB).

There is, however, a big difference between drug and vaccine in terms of the costs and benefits to subjects. The number of healthy people who have to be vaccinated is far greater than the number of TB patients who are given a course of chemotherapy: the lifetime risk of TB is of the order 0.1%–1.0% per person (Table 5.2), and yet 80% of people (i.e. 80–800 times as many) must be vaccinated. There is a small chance that anyone vaccinated would have developed TB if not vaccinated; that small benefit must be set against the risk (usually very small) of harmful side effects. In contrast, drug treatment has direct and immediate benefits for TB patients with a life-threatening disease; and it prevents the onward transmission of infection as a bonus.

BCG vaccine is effective mainly in preventing severe forms of TB in young children (meningitis and disseminated 'miliary' disease). It is sufficiently cheap (US$2–3 per dose) and safe (0.1% with moderate side effects) that it is widely recommended for children (Table 5.2).[14] Globally, an estimated 88% of 1-year-old children received BCG in 2019. But BCG does not effectively prevent lung disease in adults or stop the onward transmission of infection. If a new vaccine could be developed that is as cheap and safe as BCG, and effective in people of all ages against all forms of TB (including drug-resistant strains), it could radically change TB control, shifting the emphasis towards prevention.

Between preventive vaccination and curative drug treatment lies a third option: target people who are already infected to stop the progression to active disease. Individuals who are carrying a latent *M. tuberculosis* infection have a 1%–10% lifetime risk of progressing to TB disease (Table 5.2) so the number who must be treated prophylactically is 10–100 times the number who become TB patients. Isoniazid has high efficacy as a prophylactic drug, as well as being integral to regimens for treating active disease, but it has harmful side effects in around 1% of those treated.

In view of these trade-offs, is prevention worth the cost, effort, and potential harm, given the risk and severity of developing disease sometime in the future? This question is examined in more detail below, for vaccines and for prophylactic and curative drugs.

But there are other ways to prevent infection or to reduce the risk of TB following infection, besides vaccines and drugs. These methods target one or more of the multiple 'risk factors' for TB, such as crowding, diabetes, HIV infection, alcohol and tobacco use, and undernutrition.[10]

The weakness of this approach is that most of the modifiable risks are not very risky: they increase the chance of acquiring infection or developing disease by a factor of 2–3, and they typically exist at low prevalence in populations. So they account for a small 'attributable fraction' of TB cases and deaths, and mitigation brings small benefits. With a few exceptions (e.g. HIV in Africa, below), reducing any of these risks leads to relatively small reductions in TB cases and deaths (Table 5.1).[8]

But neutralizing these risks has benefits beyond TB control. Most of the personal and social factors listed above have other consequences for health. Therefore, as for improvements in sanitation (Chapters 2 and 7), the costs and benefits of managing them should be considered inclusively, from the

Table 5.2 The costs and benefits of various options for tuberculosis prevention and curative treatment, in view of the hazard and risks

Population	Lifetime risk TB[1] (%)	Goal of intervention	Type of intervention	Reduction in lifetime risk TB (%)	Reduction in R_0 (%)	Reduction in case fatality (%)	Costs (non-monetary)
No infection	0.1–1	Prevent infection	Vaccine	50	50	0	Moderate side effects 0.1% (if like BCG[2])
Latent infection	1–10	Prevent progression from latent to active TB	Mitigate risk	15	15	0	Variable
			Drug	50	50	0	Daily/weekly drugs 3–12 months; severe side effects drug 1%
			Vaccine	50	50	0	Moderate side effects 0.1% (if like BCG)
Active TB	100	Prevent severe disease or death; prevent transmission	Drug	0	50	90	Weeks/months of moderate/severe illness; severe side effects drug 1%

Notes:

1. Tuberculosis.

2. Bacille Calmette-Guérin.

3. These examples assume a R_0 of 2, a case fatality of untreated patients of 50%, a risk factor for TB with relative risk 2 (reduced to 1.5) and population prevalence 20%. Reductions in the lifetime risk of TB, in R_0 and in case fatality are chosen for illustration (main text).

perspective of the intervention rather than from the perspective of a specific disease (here TB).[15]

All these contingencies of risk and hazard, infection and disease, and drugs and vaccines, have been embraced by economic arguments for TB control, as follows.

The economics of tuberculosis control

Attempts to spur action on TB control by arguing that 'failure to end the epidemic is morally inexcusable and economically indefensible'[16,17] have been propagated for decades, with mixed success. On the first, a moral argument needs to be underwritten by a practical instrument—a law (stronger) or a code of conduct (weaker). Such instruments are abundant but underused. On the long list are the Universal Declaration of Human Rights and the International Covenant on Economic, Social and Cultural Rights.[18,19] Their establishment is a valuable first step, but they will only succeed through persistent efforts at implementation and enforcement, based on an understanding of the incentives for doing so.

Arguments rooted in economics have been somewhat more persuasive—but could be made even more compelling. An effort to reinvigorate health financing during the 1990s led to the landmark *World Development Report (1993), Investing in Health*.[20] That report identified TB control programmes, based on combination chemotherapy, to be one of the most cost-effective of all health interventions. At the level of each patient treated, the cost per death averted was in the range of US$75–275. At population level, adding in the extra benefit of interrupting transmission, the cost per death averted dropped to US$20–100.

These findings reinforced the World Health Organization's strategy for TB control launched in 1993 (DOTS [directly observed treatment, short course]), and they have been frequently restated.[21] In practice, TB control programmes based on drug treatment are not quite so cost-effective as first estimates suggested. In 2018, the median cost per patient treated with drug-sensitive TB was approximately US$1000 (US$973), ranging from US$100–10,000. Assuming that chemotherapy maximally reduces case fatality by 40%, from 43% to 3%, the median cost per death averted is about US$2500, about 10 times higher than suggested by *Investing in Health* (Box 2.1).

The extra benefit that should come from interrupting transmission is also in question. The onset of TB disease is often slow and coughing patients usually become infectious before they seek diagnosis and treatment, thereby transmitting infection to others. In India, the country with the largest number of new TB cases annually, the majority of patients have to navigate an unregulated market of costly and inefficient formal and informal health providers. The difficulties of early diagnosis, and therefore of interrupting transmission, explain why TB is still in slow decline (Figure 5.1). But even with these caveats, treatment as both cure and prevention is cost-effective for health services, as judged by international benchmarks (Box 2.1).

Attempts to capture the benefits of TB control in monetary terms (as cost-benefit analysis), rather than as health gains (cost-effectiveness analysis), have made big claims about the return on investment, suggesting net benefits of $10 or more for each dollar spent.[22,23] This analysis is vulnerable to two kinds of criticism. First, while the costs are cash spent, the monetary benefits are measured in terms of the value of a statistical life (VSL), which is typically estimated to be 100–150 times the average annual productivity of each person in any population, as measured by gross domestic product (GDP). This large quantity supposedly reflects the willingness to pay (through revealed preference) for a reduction in mortality, but that willingness depends on who is paying and in what context (Box 2.1).[24] Second, an estimated return on investment of 10:1 is a statistic that has little value in isolation. The point of putting monetary values on health and life is to allow a choice among different kinds of outcomes, other than health. The question, then, is whether 10:1 is a better return on investment than, say, building houses, roads, or schools.

Economic arguments notwithstanding, an essential fact of TB control is that it is hard to do in practice. In view of the persistently slow decline of the disease globally, the rest of this chapter considers the actual and perceived value of TB as a hazard; ways of amplifying the value of treatment as prevention; the potential for mitigating selected risk factors; the prospects for a high-efficacy vaccine; and the challenge of using prophylactic drug treatments more widely.

Ebola with wings

TB is perceived to be a greater threat when it behaves more like Ebola—that is, when there are relatively sudden and unexpected increases in cases or deaths, with unpredictable limits (Table 5.1; Chapter 2). The fear of adverse

change is reflected in the 'U-shaped curve of concern', a term coined when
the steady downward decline of TB in the US was abruptly reversed during
the 1980s (Figure 5.2).[25] The underlying cause was President Ronald
Reagan's withdrawal of federal funding for public services, including health
services, as the consequence of cutting taxes. The funding cuts exacerbated
poverty and overcrowding in urban areas and limited the capacity to prevent TB transmission in congregate settings, such as hospitals, prisons, and
homeless shelters. The resurgence of TB was compounded by the unavoid-
able (at the time) spread of HIV infection, which predisposed people to TB
by weakening their natural immunity to the disease.

The upswing in TB cases caused public alarm that drove political action,
and government expenditure on TB control consequently rose sharply. The
re-injection of funding, and a sense of crisis, allowed a rapid expansion of
local health department initiatives.[27] TB resumed its decline but has still

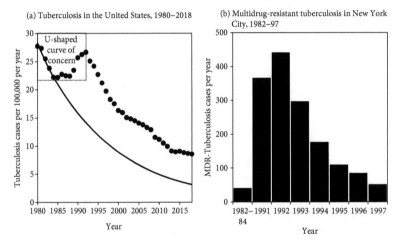

(a) Tuberculosis in the United States, 1980–2018

(b) Multidrug-resistant tuberculosis in New York City, 1982–97

Figure 5.2 The temporary failure and partial recovery of tuberculosis
(TB) control in the United States between 1980 and 2018. (a) The national
decline in TB was interrupted in 1985 (points) with additional consequences
including (b) outbreaks of multidrug-resistant TB, like that in New York
City. Since the 1985–92 failure (the upward arm of the 'U-shaped curve of
concern', inset box), the decline in TB cases has still not recovered its previous
trajectory.

Source: Data from World Health Organization. (2019). *Global tuberculosis report 2019*.
Geneva, Switzerland: World Health Organization; Frieden, T.R., Fujiwara, P.I., Washko,
R.M., Hamburg, M.A. (1995). Tuberculosis in New York City - turning the tide. *New England
Journal of Medicine*, 333: 229–33.

not recovered its earlier trajectory (Figure 5.2a). There were 243,000 excess TB cases between 1985 and 2018, a 54% increase on the number expected (the gap between points and line in Figure 5.2a). These are the cases ordinarily prevented, and which should be counted, as a benefit of routine, uninterrupted TB control programmes.

The monetary cost was also large. Direct treatment costs of the excess TB cases between 1985 and 1991 were US$340 million. Adding in the social and economic costs pushes the total up to $640 million.[28] And this was only up to 1991; the effects are still clearly visible today (Figure 5.2a). The lesson from the 1980s is that gains in TB control are hard won and easily lost, and lapses in TB control carry a large and lasting penalty.

Besides the complications of TB as an AIDS-related illness, the failure of TB control in the US during the 1980s exposed another serious problem— outbreaks of multidrug resistant TB (MDR-TB), most famously in New York City (Figure 5.2b). Suddenly, the cost of diagnosing and treating a TB case rose from hundreds to thousands of dollars, with more treatment failures and more deaths among patients. To communicate the threat, WHO characterized MDR-TB as 'Ebola with wings'.[29] The fear of resurgent TB, and in particular of emerging, untreatable forms of TB, has been a fillip to TB control around the world, spawning books such as *Timebomb: The Global Epidemic of Multi-Drug Resistant Tuberculosis*.[30] TB will never be formally designated an international health emergency (PHEIC) but, as a stimulus for action, drug-resistant TB is commonly framed as a threat to global health security.[31]

New York City was able to bring MDR-TB under control because they intervened quickly, using early case detection to cut transmission and patient supervision to achieve high cure rates. Extra effort was taken to minimize the spread of infection in hospitals, homeless shelters, and jails.[32] The intervention was probably aided by the fact that multidrug resistant strains of TB had not yet formed a large reservoir of latent infection in New York: most cases were due to recently acquired infection in the first major outbreak of MDR-TB. But the cost was high—US$1 billion to contain MDR-TB in New York City alone.

The New York experience with MDR-TB was proof of principle: drug treatment can, through cure and prevention, reverse the rise in cases and deaths from MDR-TB, even with the complications of HIV/AIDS.[33,34] During the 1990s, both the principle and the practice would need to be applied on a far greater scale, following the collapse of the Soviet Union.

Treatment for cure and prevention

The resurgence of TB in the US was overshadowed, from 1991 onwards, by the consequences of dismantling the Soviet Union (Figure 5.3). The health effects of social and economic breakdown in former Soviet countries were amply illustrated by the renewed spread of TB: between 1992 and 2004, the percentage of excess TB cases linked to the loss of GDP growth (as an indicator of social and economic impact) ranged from 38% in Estonia to 70% in Russia.[35]

In response to the crisis, Estonia acted sooner than Russia, essentially following the WHO strategy for TB control, like New York City. Since 1996 in Estonia, case incidence per 100,000 people has been halving every eight years and the mortality rate every five years (Figure 5.3). The turnaround in TB control took place later in Russia, but since 2008 the case incidence rate has been halving every thirteen years and the mortality rate every six years. The upshot is that it will have taken Russia more than three decades to return to the level of TB incidence reported in 1991, and longer still to reach the level that would have been achieved by maintaining the downward trend of the 1980s.

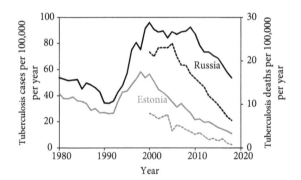

Figure 5.3 Russia (black) and Estonia (grey) suffered large surges in tuberculosis (TB) after the fall of the Soviet Union in 1991. Both countries have significantly cut TB transmission, incidence (lines) and death rates (dashes) since 2000. Estonia acted sooner than Russia; Russia has not yet returned to the case incidence rate reported in 1991.

Source: Data from World Health Organization. (2019). Global tuberculosis report 2019. Geneva, Switzerland: World Health Organization.

It is now clear that the early detection and treatment of TB can work anywhere if methodically applied and carefully adapted to local circumstances.[8] England has a far lower burden of TB than the global average, but extra effort accelerated the decline between 2011 and 2015, cutting annual incidence by 44% over that 4-year period. This result was achieved mainly through interventions targeted to immigrants from high-burden countries: pre-entry screening for TB, plus the diagnosis and treatment of latent TB infection.[36] In 2018, the number of TB cases in England was the lowest ever recorded.[37]

P is for prevention, much better than cure

So runs the first line of the children's 'Preventorium' song (R is for rest in the open pure air, and so on).[38] Created in the US in the early 1900s, preventoria were institutions, mainly for pre-tubercular children—they were at risk of TB but did not yet have the disease (unlike sanatoria, which were for the sick). Before there were any drugs and vaccines, preventoria aimed to protect their patients from infection and disease, and stop the transmission of infection to others. They did this by means that were thought to be effective at the time: isolation, rest and supervised exercise, nutritious food, physical and personal hygiene, and exposure to fresh air and sunshine, often in pastoral settings such as woods and forests, or near oceans, rivers, and lakes.[39]

Preventoria were conceived with a limited understanding of the factors that affect the risk of TB. Another century of epidemiological studies has led to the discovery of a wide range of biological, behavioural, social, and economic factors that affect the risk of TB. But most of these factors are relatively low risk and, even when highly prevalent, account for a minority of TB cases.[8] Consequently, reducing exposure to these factors across whole populations, including people at low and high risk, is not expected to have a big impact on TB.[40] This is why TB declined slowly in Europe and North America in the first half of the twentieth century, before the discovery of anti-tuberculosis drugs in the 1940s (Chapter 1).

There is, however, a more powerful argument for modifying these risks: all of them have broader consequences for health. People who are undernourished (low body mass index) are at three times the risk of TB, and undernutrition accounts for an estimated 19% of TB worldwide.[10] In areas of the world with a high prevalence of undernutrition, such as the central eastern states of India, dietary improvements have multiple benefits, in addition to reducing the risk of TB.[41,42] Better nutrition for children and adults restores energy deficits, increases resistance to other infectious diseases, and improves survival rates.

Underweight is one form of malnutrition; overweight is another. Type 2 diabetes linked to high body mass index has become a global pandemic, currently affecting more than 400 million people worldwide.[43] Diabetes patients have a higher chance of developing TB (50% increase in risk), with the result that 360,000 TB cases and 40,000 TB deaths are attributable to diabetes each year.[10] Diabetes is not the main driving force for TB in any population: a comparison of the contrasting forces driving TB in India (high TB burden) and the Republic of Korea (low TB burden) found demographic processes to be far more important: population growth in India and population aging in Korea.[15] But the link between TB and diabetes is strong enough to recommend screening both ways: diabetes tests should be part of the care provided to TB patients; and diabetes patients should be examined for, and educated about, signs of TB.[44,45] The joint care of patients with TB, diabetes, and other disorders linked to malnutrition potentially yields greater benefits per unit cost in integrated health services.

Bigger reductions in TB can be obtained by targeting factors that are high risk for individuals, and highly prevalent in populations. The best example is ART used to treat HIV/AIDS in sub-Saharan Africa. ART restores immunity in general, and specifically against *M. tuberculosis*, and halts the progression from TB infection to disease. Whereas diabetes and undernutrition increase the risk of TB two- to three-fold, people infected with HIV have a 15-fold risk. In Botswana, for example, the prevalence of HIV infection was 24% on average between 2003 and 2016, and an estimated 77% was attributable to HIV co-infection. Given the high risk and prevalence of HIV, ART is a powerful tool for TB control. Although the use of ART varied among African countries over the period 2003–16, ART prevented an estimated 30% of all the TB that would have occurred in 12 countries: 1.88 million episodes of illness in total (Figure 5.4).[46]

The differences in ART uptake between African countries prompt deeper questions about the motives for treatment and prevention—why the coverage of ART was higher, for example, in Botswana than in South Africa. Botswana's comparative success has a cultural and historical context, set by Twsana tribal leadership: since independence in 1966, successive governments have invested in public institutions, policies, and services to tackle ill health and poverty.[47,48] Botswana was the first African country to provide ART free of charge to everyone who needed it. In contrast, South

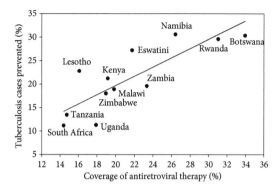

Figure 5.4 Association between the coverage of antiretroviral treatment and the prevention of tuberculosis cases among people infected with HIV for 12 countries in sub-Saharan Africa, 2003–16.

Adapted under a Creative Commons Attribution 3.0 IGO (CC BY 3.0 IGO) from Dye, C., Williams, B.G. (2019). Tuberculosis decline in populations affected by HIV: a retrospective study of 12 countries in the WHO African Region. *Bulletin of the World Health Organization*, 97: 405–14.

Africa's earliest efforts to contain HIV/AIDS were hijacked by a dispute over whether AIDS was caused by HIV infection. South Africa was consequently slower to expand treatment, but now has the largest number of people on ART worldwide, and the largest number of people on isoniazid preventive therapy for TB (below). In 2015, South Africa also became the first country in sub-Saharan Africa to give full regulatory approval for pre-exposure prophylaxis (PreP), using ART to protect people from acquiring HIV infection, and therefore from TB too.[46] The wider lesson from these experiences in Botswana and South Africa is that public health practitioners generally benefit from understanding domestic, legal, regulatory, and policy frameworks, and the cultural foundations of these norms.[19]

From the perspective of TB, ART is a drug treatment to manage a major risk. Other technologies are available to prevent TB directly: vaccines, and prophylactic drugs to neutralize latent *M. tuberculosis* infection, as follows.

Vaccines: Preventing infection and disease

A high efficacy vaccine could transform TB control, shifting the emphasis further towards prevention, reducing the need for combination chemotherapy.

Endemic infectious diseases, such as malaria, TB, and HIV/AIDS, persist partly because it is technically difficult to make better tools for prevention—especially vaccines. None of the pathogens that cause these diseases (protozoan, bacteria, virus) stimulate long-lasting immunity to first or subsequent infections, and few vaccines are more efficacious than natural immunity to infection (*Haemophilus influenzae*, a cause of bacterial pneumonia, and rabies are examples). In the development of TB disease, immunity actually conspires with infection to create lung cavities from which bacteria are expelled by coughing.

Although investment in TB vaccine research increased little over the period 2010–18 (around US$100 million per year),[11] coordinated international efforts have increased the momentum of vaccine discovery.[49–51] Among the most promising candidates is M72/AS01E, a 'subunit' vaccine that presents a specific, synthesized antigen to the immune system. In clinical trials, M72/AS01E safely prevented TB in 54% of adults carrying latent infections.[55] Given the disappointing history of TB vaccination, this result is a breakthrough.[52] However, this vaccine alone would not prevent a large number of TB cases quickly. An estimated 1.7 billion people carry latent infection;[9] and they contribute to about 13% of all TB cases arising each year. M72/AS01E would cut that percentage to 6%. There is also the challenge of vaccinating a large number of adults, for whom there are no routine vaccine delivery mechanisms (unlike for children; though COVID-19 may change that).

While the search for new vaccines continues, there is renewed interest in finding extra life in the old ones. One option is BCG revaccination, given as a booster for adolescents as they move into adulthood, the period of highest risk for pulmonary disease.[54] Another promising discovery is that BCG has high efficacy, at least in macaques, when given intravenously (IV), directly into the bloodstream rather than into skin or muscle.[55] The question now is whether IV injection is safe and efficacious for humans, and practical on a large scale.

It might be optimistic to suggest that a new vaccine is imminent[51] but the pipeline is now fuller than ever before: 14 candidates were in clinical trials as of April 2020.[10] As a comparative measure of urgency, 32 candidate COVID-19 vaccines had entered clinical trials by the end of August 2020, within nine months of the emergence of the new coronavirus. Hundreds more are being added to the COVID-19 R&D pipeline.

Preventive therapy: Avoiding harm and limiting risk

In the search for a new mode of vaccination, the main challenge is to raise efficacy without compromising safety. The problem for prophylactic drug treatment is different: we already have high-efficacy drugs; the task is to improve uptake by reducing the cost, duration, and potential harm of treatment.[56]

A course of isoniazid, taken daily for nine months, gives more than 90% protection against TB to people who are already (latently) infected with *M. tuberculosis*. The hitch is that few healthy people, who are generally at low risk of developing TB disease, are willing to take a drug daily for nine months, especially when there is a risk of harmful side effects.

The side effects of isoniazid include nausea, vomiting, and peripheral neuropathy, but the most severe is liver injury at a frequency of around 1% (higher in older people), with occasional fatalities. For comparison, the life-time risk of TB among people carrying a latent infection is also of the order of 1%.[57] In other words, the chance of preventing TB is about the same as the risk of harmful side effects, a disincentive for prevention.

In view of the costs and benefits of isoniazid preventive therapy, it is not surprising that the uptake is low: 350,000 children under 5 years old, house-hold contacts of TB patients, started preventive therapy in 2018—only 27% of those eligible.[5] Preventive therapy protects HIV-positive people from TB, but the impact on the epidemic has so far been much less than that of ART (Figure 5.4).[49] There are a small number of other potential benefi-ciaries: people who have weakened immunity due to another health condi-tion (e.g. gold miners with silicosis), or because of medical treatment (e.g. tumour necrosis factor [TNF]-α inhibitors that prevent inflammation due to arthritis; organ transplants).[58]

Preventive therapy is likely to achieve higher coverage, with greater ef-fects on TB epidemics, given shorter, safer, low-cost drug regimens, which can be targeted at those at high risk. One of the front-runners is a three-month regimen of once-weekly isoniazid plus rifapentine (in the same group of drugs as rifampicin). This appears to be as efficacious as nine months of isoniazid but with a lower risk of liver toxicity and higher rates of treatment completion.[56, 59]

Tuberculosis drugs have now been available for 70 years, but they are still not used to their full potential—to prevent transmission in addition to curing illness and reducing mortality. This is partly because diagnosis is late and drug treatment is difficult to administer. New technologies that are easier to use would give extra impetus to TB control: a household diagnostic test, a short-course prophylactic or curative drug, or a more efficacious vaccine. If BCG could be replaced with a vaccine as efficacious as those for polio or smallpox, then we could begin to contemplate TB eradication.

Summary

Familiar endemic diseases such as TB are rarely seen as health emergencies, even though they kill millions of people each year. This chapter describes a variety of ways to remedy the neglect, illustrated by TB, including: highlight new dangers from old hazards, such as the emergence of multi-drug resistant strains; eliminate the prevention–cure dichotomy by exploiting the benefits of 'treatment as prevention', when drugs that cure illness also prevent the transmission of infection to others; neutralize major risks for TB, such as co-infection with human immunodeficiency virus (HIV), in settings where these risks cause a high proportion of cases and deaths; and mitigate the large number of weaker TB risks that have benefits for other health conditions (diabetes, undernutrition) and for society more widely (homelessness, crowding). This wider context aligns the specific aims of neglected disease control with the larger goals of Universal Health Coverage and the Agenda for Sustainable Development.

References

1. TB Alliance. TB is a pandemic. 2019. https://www.tballiance.org/why-new-tb-drugs/global-pandemic (accessed 7 January 2021).
2. Institute for Health Metrics and Evaluation (IHME). GBD Results Tool. 2020. http://ghdx.healthdata.org/gbd-results-tool (accessed 7 January 2021).
3. Plotkin BJ, Hardiman MC. The international health regulations (2005), tuberculosis and air travel. *Travel Medicine and Infectious Diseases* 2010; *8*: 9.
4. World Health Organization. Neglected tropical diseases. 2019 (accessed 12 December 2019).
5. Stop TB Partnership. *Global Plan to End TB: 2018–2022*. Geneva: Stop TB Partnership; 2019. 12.9.
6. Global Burden of Disease Health Financing Collaborator Network. Health sector spending and spending on HIV/AIDS, tuberculosis, and malaria, and development assistance for health: Progress towards Sustainable Development Goal 3. *Lancet* 2020; *396*: 693–724.

7. The Global Fund. Financials. 2020. https://www.theglobalfund.org/en/financials (accessed 7 January 2021).
8. Dye C. *The Population Biology of Tuberculosis.* Princeton: Princeton University Press; 2015.
9. Houben RM, Dodd PJ. The global burden of latent tuberculosis infection: A reestimation using mathematical modelling. *PLoS Medicine* 2016; *13*: e1002152.
10. World Health Organization. *Global Tuberculosis Report 2019.* Geneva: World Health Organization; 2020.
11. Treatment Action Group. *Tuberculosis Research Funding Trends, 2005–2018.* New York: Treatment Action Group; 2019.
12. World Health Organization. *Progress towards Achieving Global Tuberculosis Targets and Implementation of the UN Political Declaration on Tuberculosis.* Geneva: World Health Organization; 2020.
13. Keeling MJ, Rohani P. *Modeling Infectious Diseases in Humans and Animals.* Princeton: Princeton University Press; 2008.
14. Bourdin Trunz B, Fine PEM, Dye C. Effect of BCG vaccination on childhood tuberculous meningitis and miliary tuberculosis: A meta-analysis and assessment of cost-effectiveness. *Lancet* 2006; *367*: 1175–82.
15. Dye C, Bourdin Trunz B, Lönnroth K, Roglic G, Williams BG. Nutrition, diabetes and tuberculosis in the epidemiological transition. *PLoS One* 2011; *6*: e21161.
16. Reid MJA, Arinaminpathy N, Bloom A, et al. Building a tuberculosis-free world: The Lancet Commission on tuberculosis. *Lancet* 2019; *393*: 1331–84.
17. Reid MJA, Goosby E. A tuberculosis-free world: Is it a delusion?—Authors' reply. *Lancet* 2019; *394*: 913–4.
18. Stop TB Partnership. *The Declaration of the Rights of People Affected by Tuberculosis.* Geneva: Stop TB Partnership; 2019.
19. Verani AR, Emerson CN, Lederer P, et al. The role of the law in reducing tuberculosis transmission in Botswana, South Africa and Zambia. *Bulletin of the World Health Organization* 2016; *94*: 415–23.
20. World Bank. *World Development Report 1993: Investing in Health.* New York: Oxford University Press; 1993.
21. Jamison D, Gelband H, Horton S, et al. DCP3: Disease Control Priorities. 2018. http://dcp-3.org (accessed 7 January 2021).
22. Laxminarayan R, Klein E, Dye C, Floyd K, Darley S, Odeyi O. *Economic Benefit of Tuberculosis Control.* Washington DC: World Bank; 2007.
23. Bloom B, Atun R, Cohen T, et al. Tuberculosis. In: Jamison DT, ed. *Disease Control Priorities.* 3rd edn. Washington, DC: Oxford University Press; 2017: 233–313.
24. US Environmental Protection Agency (USEPA). *Guidelines for Preparing Economic Analyses.* Washington, DC: USEPA, Office of the Administrator; 2000.
25. Reichman LB. The U-shaped curve of concern. *American Review of Respiratory Disease* 1991; *144*: 741–2.
26. Frieden TR, Fujiwara PI, Washko RM, Hamburg MA. Tuberculosis in New York City—Turning the tide. *New England Journal of Medicine* 1995; *333*: 229–33.

27. Bayer R, Dupuis L. Tuberculosis, public health, and civil liberties. *Annual Review of Public Health* 1995; *16*: 307–26.
28. Bloom BR, Murray CJL. Tuberculosis: Commentary on a reemergent killer. *Science* 1992; *257*: 1055–64.
29. Voelker R. Ebola with wings. *JAMA* 1998; *280*: 1216.
30. Reichman LB, Tanne, J.H. *Timebomb: The Global Epidemic of Multi-Drug Resistant Tuberculosis*. New York: McGraw-Hill; 2001.
31. Kenyon T. Tuberculosis is a threat to global health security. *Health Affairs (Millwood)* 2018; *37*: 1536.
32. Frieden TR, Woodley CL, Crawford JT, Lew D, Dooley SM. The molecular epidemiology of tuberculosis in New York City: The importance of nosocomial transmission and laboratory error. *Tubercle and Lung Disease* 1996; *77*: 407–13.
33. Dye C, Williams BG. Slow elimination of multidrug-resistant tuberculosis. *Science Translational Medicine* 2009; *1*: 3ra8.
34. Dye C. Doomsday postponed? Preventing and reversing epidemics of drug-resistant tuberculosis *Nature Reviews Microbiology* 2009; *10*: 81–7.
35. Arinaminpathy N, Dye C. Health in financial crises: Economic recession and tuberculosis in Central and Eastern Europe. *Journal of the Royal Society Interface* 2010; *7*: 1559–69.
36. Thomas HL, Harris RJ, Muzyamba MC, et al. Reduction in tuberculosis incidence in the UK from 2011 to 2015: A population-based study. *Thorax* 2018; *73*: 769–75.
37. Public Health England. Tuberculosis in England: 2020 report. https://assets.publishing.service.gov.uk/government/uploads/system/uploads/attachment_data/file/943356/TB_Annual_Report_2020.pdf (accessed 7 January 2021).
38. Bynum H. *Spitting Blood*. Oxford: Oxford University Press; 2012.
39. Grose MJ. Landscape and children's health: Old natures and new challenges for the preventorium. *Health & Place* 2011; *17*: 94–102.
40. Lonnroth K, Weil DE. Mass prophylaxis of tuberculosis through social protection. *Lancet Infect Diseases* 2014; *14*: 1032–4.
41. Oxlade O, Murray M. Tuberculosis and poverty: Why are the poor at greater risk in India? *PloS one* 2012; *11*: e47533.
42. Oxlade O, Huang CC, Murray M. Estimating the impact of reducing undernutrition on the tuberculosis epidemic in the central eastern states of India: A dynamic modeling study. *PloS one* 2015; *10*: e0128187.
43. NCD Risk Factor Collaboration. Worldwide trends in diabetes since 1980: A pooled analysis of 751 population-based studies with 4.4 million participants. *Lancet* 2016; *387*: 1513–30.
44. Lönnroth K, Williams BG, Cegielski P, Dye C. A consistent log-linear relationship between tuberculosis incidence and body mass index. *International Journal of Epidemiology* 2010; *39*: 149–55.
45. Lin Y, Harries AD, Kumar AMV, et al. *Management of Diabetes-Tuberculosis: A Guide to the Essential Practice*. Paris: International Union Against Tuberculosis and Lung Disease; 2019.

46. Dye C, Williams BG. Tuberculosis decline in populations affected by HIV: A retrospective study of 12 countries in the WHO African Region. *Bulletin of the World Health Organization* 2019; *97*: 405–14.

47. Acemoglu D, Johnson S, Robinson JA. An African success story: Botswana. In: Rodrik D, ed. *In Search of Prosperity: Analytic Narratives on Economic Growth*. Princeton: Princeton University Press; 2003: 80–119.

48. Acemoglu D, Robinson JA. *Why Nations Fail: The Origins of Power, Prosperity and Poverty*. New York: Crown Publishing Group; 2012.

49. TuBerculosis Vaccine Initiative (TBVI). TuBerculosis Vaccine Initiative. www.tbvi.eu (accessed 7 January 2021).

50. Porcelli SA, Jacobs WR, Jr. Exacting Edward Jenner's revenge: The quest for a new tuberculosis vaccine. *Science Translational Medicine* 2019; *11*: eaax4219.

51. Andersen P, Scriba TJ. Moving tuberculosis vaccines from theory to practice. *Nature Reviews Immunology* 2019; *19*: 550–62.

52. Van Der Meeren O, Hatherill M, Nduba V, et al. Phase 2b controlled trial of M72/AS01E vaccine to prevent tuberculosis. *New England Journal of Medicine* 2018; *379*: 1621–34.

53. World Health Organization. Tuberculosis vaccine development. 2020. https://www.who.int/immunization/research/development/tuberculosis/en/ (accessed 7 January 2021).

54. Dye C. Making wider use of the world's most widely-used vaccine: BCG revaccination reconsidered. *Journal of the Royal Society Interface* 2013; *10*: 20130365.

55. Darrah PA, Zeppa JJ, Maiello P, et al. Prevention of tuberculosis in macaques after intravenous BCG immunization. *Nature* 2020; *577*: 95–102.

56. Getahun H, Matteelli A, Chaisson RE, Raviglione M. Latent Mycobacterium tuberculosis infection. *New England Journal of Medicine* 2015; *372*: 2127–35.

57. Horsburgh CR, Jr., O'Donnell M, Chamblee S, et al. Revisiting rates of reactivation tuberculosis: A population-based approach. *American Journal of Respiratory and Critical Care Medicine* 2010; *182*: 420–5.

58. Churchyard GJ, Swindells S. Controlling latent TB tuberculosis infection in high-burden countries: A neglected strategy to end TB. *PLoS Medicine* 2019; *16*: e1002787.

59. Matteelli A, Sulis G, Capone S, D'Ambrosio L, Migliori GB, Getahun H. Tuberculosis elimination and the challenge of latent tuberculosis. *Presse Med* 2017; *46*: e13–e21.

6

The burden of choice

The sugar tax [is] a vicious tax because it [is] a tax on the food of the people.

Harold Cox, Labour MP for Preston
(*The Guardian*, 10 July 1907)

Sound, general advice on healthy living—how to reduce the risk of heart disease, stroke, cancers, and diabetes—is uncontroversial among medical experts: eat a varied and balanced diet, get enough sleep, exercise often, don't smoke, drink alcohol in moderation. And follow all of this advice, not just part of it. Such guidance is now widely available,[1] although distorted by powerful manufacturers with a heavy sales pitch and by the promoters of misinformed goop.

Once the good advice has been separated from the bad, the next task is to follow it. Since the immediate benefits of unhealthy choices appear to exceed the longer-term costs, neither the consumers nor the purveyors of toxic substances are inclined to self-restraint. For consumers, prevention is compromised because today's habitual, socially acceptable pleasures (alcohol, tobacco, salt, sugar, and others) outweigh the risk of poor health acquired incrementally, with the worst consequences expected in the distant, devalued future.

Ultimately, lifestyle choices rest with consumers, and even the most addictive unhealthy behaviours might eventually change through individual choice alone. However, the burden of choice on consumers is lighter when shared and governments, in particular, have the motives, means, and powers to intervene between commercial supply and consumer demand. 'Behaviour' invariably refers to what consumers do, and yet the behaviours of governments and commercial suppliers are critical too.

The Great Health Dilemma. Christopher Dye, Oxford University Press. © Oxford University Press 2021.
DOI: 10.1093/oso/9780198853824.003.0006

Nanny states

James Baldwin[2] elegantly stated the consumer's predicament: 'People pay for what they do, and still more for what they have allowed themselves to become. And they pay for it very simply: by the lives they lead.'

But elected governments are there to help people lead better lives. Governments, unlike most consumers, have access to the most accurate information. They know that the burden of illness on populations and health services, due to unhealthy behaviours, is certain, quantifiable, and already large, and that they must cover at least part of the cost. They also have at their disposal some of the most powerful preventive mechanisms— taxation (alcohol and tobacco) and regulation (e.g. mandatory salt limits in food, banning trans fats), plus subsidies and services, that can be used to encourage the use of preventive methods (e.g. antihypertensive drugs to cut the risk of heart attack and stroke). The first of these, excise taxes on consumer goods (and 'bads') can actually raise revenue for governments. Taxing bads is also a way of relieving taxes on other forms of wealth, such as savings and income.[3]

Adam Smith himself was clear on the opportunities for state intervention. In 1776 he wrote: 'Sugar, rum and tobacco are commodities which are nowhere necessaries of life ... and which are therefore extremely proper subjects of taxation.'[4] However, government proposals to tax and regulate dangerous substances, as part of a strategy for prevention,[5] invariably spark debate about the boundaries between individual and collective responsibility.[6] Those who emphasize personal responsibility decry control by the 'nanny state'. Those who favour intervention argue that responsibility must be commensurate with the freedom to choose. Those who are most disadvantaged, and who stand to gain most from intervention, are least able to choose. In this view, the notion of tax as the wage of sin ('sin tax') is inappropriate: taxation is not an imposition; rather, it is part of the social contract between citizens and government, an agreed way of helping consumers to make healthier choices. It is one way of creating the 'fully engaged' population imagined by Derek Wanless, aligning incentives for collective action (Chapter 3).[7] It is also a pathway to health equity.

Given the different preferences and powers of consumers, manufacturers, and governments, this chapter explores the options for limiting two of Adam Smith's unnecessary commodities: tobacco and sugar. The first step is to put both of these health hazards in a wider context—in relation to the burden and control of non-communicable diseases.

Non-communicable diseases and their causes

The great majority of people around the world now die from non-communicable diseases and injuries, rather than from infections. Among 57 million deaths in 2017, 42 million were from non-communicable conditions including, in rank order, ischaemic (coronary) heart disease, stroke, chronic obstructive lung disease, dementia, cancers of airways (trachea, bronchus, and lung), diabetes, and road accidents.[8]

The risks underlying these causes have been classified as behavioural (21.6 million deaths e.g. alcohol, tobacco, sugar, salt, vitamins, and others), metabolic (18.6 million e.g. high blood pressure, blood sugar, body mass index), and environmental and occupational (11.3 million e.g. air pollution, exposure to carcinogens). Global trends in death rates attributable to these risks vary greatly. The death rate linked to household air pollution is falling but is persistently high for ambient (outdoor) particulate matter pollution; vitamin A deficiency is in rapid decline but high body mass index has been more refractory to change; tobacco use is falling, albeit slowly, but the use of illicit drugs is not (Figure 6.1).[9]

The benefits of prevention for health depend on the link between risk and disease. Wherever there is a major risk to health, it is a target for intervention. Cancer trends among men and women in Scotland illustrate the point (Figure 6.2). The risk of malignant skin cancer (melanoma) can be reduced by limiting exposure to ultra-violet light, and yet incidence and death rates have been rising since the early 1990s. The chances of surviving lung cancer are poor, but most lung cancers are due to tobacco use. Quitting smoking is the best way to prevent lung cancer. The per capita incidence of breast cancer, the most frequent cancer among women in Scotland, has been rising, and not only because the female population is aging. Unlike lung cancer, there is no single dominant, modifiable risk for breast cancer. The factors affecting risk are weak and numerous, and some are not easily modifiable: older maternal age at the birth of a first child, fewer children, post-menopausal obesity, and alcohol use. However, survival rates are improving, probably due to earlier diagnosis and more rapid treatment (cure rather than prevention). Cases of colorectal cancer are in slow decline, and mortality is falling faster still. These trends are probably due to better prevention and cure—a decline in exposure to risks, plus earlier diagnosis (via the Scottish Bowel Screening Programme, removal of pre-malignant polyps at colonoscopies) and advances in treatment.[10,11]

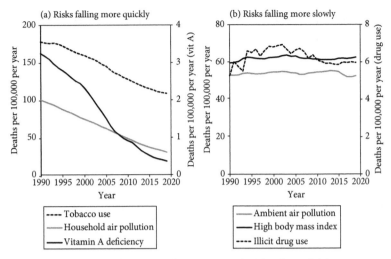

Figure 6.1 Global trends in mortality associated with selected risks to health. The graphs compare risks that are falling (a) relatively quickly or (b) slowly: vitamin A deficiency and high body mass index (BMI ≥ 25, black lines), household air and ambient particulate matter pollution (grey lines), tobacco and illicit drug use.

Source: Data from Institute for Health Metrics and Evaluation (IHME). GBD Compare - Viz Hub. 2020.

Tobacco: Legalized harm

Tobacco users trade short-term satisfaction for long-term harm. The satisfaction might be measured by the six trillion cigarettes still smoked each year; the harm by the 100 million people killed by tobacco during the twentieth century, about the same number as died of tuberculosis (Chapter 5). If present trends continue, tobacco will kill one billion people in the twenty-first century. Worldwide, about 1 in 5 of all people (1.3 billion) still use tobacco, mostly men (1.1 billion).[12–14]

Globally, the proportion of people who use tobacco is falling, and so is the number of smoking-related deaths per capita (Figure 6.1). But the total number of smokers is barely in decline: continued population growth, coupled with the income growth that makes cigarettes more affordable in developing countries (Figure 2.3),[15] means that the number of smokers is expected to remain over a billion well beyond 2025.

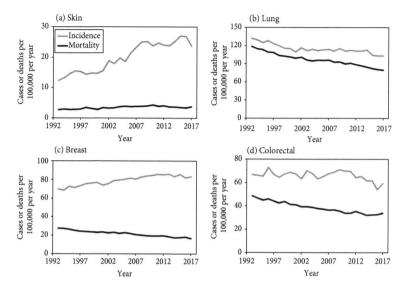

Figure 6.2 Trends in incidence and mortality (age standardized rates) from four groups of cancers among men and women in Scotland (both sexes combined).

Source: Data from National Statistics (Information Services Division). Cancer Incidence and Prevalence in Scotland (to December 2017). Edinburgh: National Statistics (Information Services Division), 2019; National Statistics (Information Services Division). Cancer Mortality in Scotland (2017). Edinburgh: National Statistics (Information Services Division), 2019.

Most smokers are aware of the risk of developing one or more chronic or fatal diseases, including bronchitis, emphysema, and more than a dozen forms of cancer. Some will also be aware that the life expectancy of regular smokers is shorter (by at least 10 years) than for non-smokers and that smoking causes the majority of deaths (up to two-thirds) in people who continue to smoke.[16]

But hundreds of millions of people continue to smoke, suck, chew, and snuff tobacco because it is addictively pleasurable. Even if there is a high risk of dying from a smoking-related illness, that outcome, for a young adult, is not immediate.[17,18] Some smokers may prefer to postpone the pain of escaping the addiction: quitting before the age of 40 cuts the risk of dying from a smoking-related disease by about 90% (compared with continuing to smoke beyond 40).[19]

The health risks linked to smoking also have to be put in the broader context of livelihoods and lifestyles. Whereas health services usually consider smoking and its consequences separately from other health risks, individuals are more likely to place tobacco harms among life's other adversities. One sign of this, within a country or community, is that the prevalence of smoking tends to be higher among people who are more socially and economically disadvantaged, even though the cost of tobacco is a higher fraction of their income (Figure 6.3).[20–22] Tobacco appears to magnify health inequality via social and economic inequality.

As smokers become aware of the harms caused by tobacco, most want to quit.[19,23,24] The burden of making that choice—shifting the balance of costs and benefits—can be lightened by helping them to do so. The measures known to be effective are the basis of the Framework Convention on Tobacco Control (the only modern international treaty in public health), implemented via the World Health Organization's (WHO) MPOWER strategy: Monitor tobacco use and prevention policies, Protect people from smoke, Offer help to quit, Warn about the dangers, Enforce bans on advertising, and Raise taxes on tobacco.[23–27]

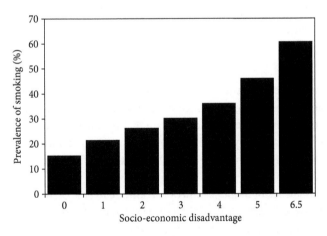

Figure 6.3 Variation in the prevalence of tobacco smoking with social and economic disadvantage (higher score on horizontal axis). Data are from a survey of 88,000 adults aged 16 or over in England, 2001–08.

Source: Data from Hiscock, R., Bauld, L., Amos, A., Platt, S. (2012). Smoking and socioeconomic status in England: the rise of the never smoker and the disadvantaged smoker. *Journal of Public Health* (Oxford), 34: 390–6.

The last of these mechanisms, taxation, is potentially the most powerful. Tobacco taxes cut consumption and raise revenue for governments wherever they have been applied around the world.[2,13,28,29] The government of France, for example, increased cigarette excise taxes substantially from the early 1990s onwards, tripling cigarette prices in real terms by 2010. Cigarette consumption dropped and so did the death rate from lung cancer (Figure 6.4).[13,30,31] There is an inverse relationship between death and taxes. Taxing specific commodities, like tobacco, can rapidly deliver health benefits in any country, irrespective of national wealth and other forms of taxation. The Philippines raised tax on all types of cigarettes more than fourfold in 2012. Prices of the cheapest, most popular brands rose by more than 50%. Between 2011 and 2015, tobacco-tax revenues more than doubled, and the smoking rate among adults fell from 30% to 25%.[32] Tax revenues were used to help finance the expansion of health services in the Philippines.[19]

In general, taxes are more effective in countries where the price of tobacco makes up a larger fraction of income. Across the European Union, countries with a gross national income per capita lower than US$5,400 were more responsive to taxation (high price 'elasticity') than those with

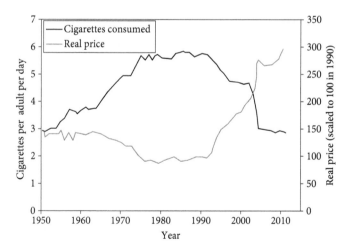

Figure 6.4 Changes in the inflation-adjusted price of cigarettes (scaled to 100 in 1990, grey line) and in cigarette consumption (of cigarettes per adult per day, black line) in France, 1950–2011.

Reproduced under a Creative Commons Attribution 3.0 IGO (CC BY 3.0 IGO) from Gelband, H., P. Jha, R. Sankaranarayanan, and S. Horton (Eds). (2015). *Cancer Disease Control Priorities*, third edition, volume 3. Washington, DC, USA: World Bank.

incomes above this threshold.[15] Wealthier people are less sensitive to price but more aware of the risks to their health and the benefits of stopping. They are therefore more inclined to stop smoking by choice.

This points to a complementary approach to tobacco control—offering carrots while wielding sticks. Most of the instruments used to discourage smoking—prohibitions, taxes, regulations, and cautions—are prevention by punishment and threat. They warn of future health lost (from lung cancer, etc.) rather than advertising the benefits of good health gained.

How the risk of poor health later is balanced against the chance of better health sooner is a topic for behavioural research (Chapter 2). However, smokers should be aware that health quickly recovers after giving up cigarettes. Within 20 minutes of the last cigarette, heart rate and blood pressure begin to fall. Within 12 hours, carbon monoxide in the blood drops to normal levels. After 2–12 weeks, blood circulation and lung function improve. After 1–9 months, coughing and shortness of breath subside. After one year, the risk of coronary heart disease is about half that of a smoker. After 5–15 years, the risk of death due to heart disease is halved, and the risk of stroke is the same as for a non-smoker. After 15 years, the risk of coronary heart disease is no greater than for someone who never smoked.[33]

Sugar: Surplus pleasure

In *The Saccharine Disease* (1974), T.L. Cleave considered how members of the public might balance the pros and cons of eating and drinking refined carbohydrates. He guessed that 'in prevention, very little; in treatment, quite a lot; in short, people will go on enjoying themselves till they get hurt.'[34]

Sugars added to food and drinks by manufacturers and consumers, plus sugars naturally present in honey, syrups, and fruit juices, push up the energy content of what we eat. Consuming free sugars compromises the quality of a diet by providing energy without protein, fibre, minerals, and vitamins. Excess energy from sugar often leads to unhealthy weight gain and a higher risk of obesity.[35] Overweight and obesity are associated, more or less strongly, with type II diabetes, cancers, cardiovascular diseases, depression, and social stigmatization.[36–38]

The human body is a calorie trap: it efficiently stores excess energy as fat, and then obstinately defends its removal.[39] In this sense, it is physiologically easier to prevent weight gain than to reverse it. Nevertheless, if obese people can lose weight and become physically active, they can reduce the risk of metabolic diseases such as diabetes.[40]

Like tobacco, sweet food is a source of instant gratification. Unlike tobacco, sugar is not harmful per se, only when consumed in excess, especially as part of a poor diet. Eating it is not socially unacceptable, nor does it pose an immediate hazard to others. Because sugar is toxic only in quantity, its consumption is harder to control than tobacco.

Like cigarette smokers, most consumers of unhealthy foods want help to resist temptation. The forms of help known to be effective include price increases in restaurants, shops, and leisure centres; labels that are easy to understand; promotion and better placement of healthier drinks in supermarkets; government food benefits (e.g. food stamps) that exclude sugary drinks; community campaigns focused on supporting healthy choices; and schemes to make low-calorie drinks, especially water, more readily available in homes, schools, and restaurants.[41]

As for tobacco, sugar taxes work but need careful design and experimental calibration. Flat-rate taxes aim to deter the consumption of sugary drinks; tiered tax mechanisms also encourage manufacturers to reformulate beverages with lower sugar content beneath tax thresholds, so they pay less tax or no tax at all.[42] Some nutritionists contend that it is preferable to tax sugar itself rather than, say, sugary drinks by volume: the tax should be proportional to the harm caused.[43]

In April 2018, the UK government introduced the Soft Drinks Industry Levy (SDIL) as one approach to tackling childhood obesity.[44,45] As a result, the total amount of sugar sold in soft drinks in the UK was reduced by 29% in 2018, as compared with 2015. Three-quarters (73%) of the reduction was due to reformulation of existing products by manufacturers or the introduction of new, low-sugar drinks; 27% was due to changes in consumer purchasing behaviour.[46]

By mid-2019, 42 countries worldwide, from India to Ireland and South Africa to Sri Lanka, had levied taxes on sugar-sweetened beverages through a mix of tax mechanisms—excise or value-added taxes, and based on volume or sugar content.[34,43,47,48]

If taxes on sugar-sweetened drinks are effective, why not tax sugary snacks too? High-sugar snacks (confectionery) usually provide more free sugar and energy than sugar-sweetened beverages.

Consumers are sensitive to price increases in foods, including sugar-sweetened foods, just as they are for drinks. Countries, including Mexico, Finland, and Hungary have introduced taxes on sugary snacks, among other unhealthy foods. In Mexico, all 'non-essential' foods with 275 or more kcal/100g are taxed at 8%, including confectionery such as biscuits, chocolate, and cereal bars. The effect has been to reduce purchases by 5%–6%, with greater effects among those who habitually bought more sweets.[49] Exploring what might be achieved in the UK, one evaluation found that a 20% price increase could reduce the prevalence of obesity by 2.7% in a year, with bigger than average effects among obese people in low-income households.[49] It also concluded that the health benefits of taxing high-sugar snacks would be greater than from comparable price increases on sugary drinks, because the foods contain more sugar than the drinks.

Whereas taxes on the price of goods discourage supply and demand, guidelines and voluntary codes of conduct for manufacturers and consumers are generally ineffective. Public Health England developed a voluntary programme in which manufacturers would cut sugar in snacks, with poor results.[50] Commercial producers were asked to reduce the sugar content of a range of foods by 20% over the period 2016–20. The net reduction in sugar content was only 2.9% after two years and the consumption of some products was pushed up by promotional offers and advertising. Some food manufacturers actually increased the sugar content of their products.

The mix of legislation and guidance in the UK has generated few positive results over the past decade. Between 2011 and 2019, the prevalence of obesity in 10–11-year-old children in England remained stable at about 20%.[51] Aware of the slow progress, the UK government announced, in July 2020, a new plan to tackle obesity in children and adults. Extra impetus came from evidence that people who are overweight and suffering from COVID-19 are more likely to be admitted to hospital, and more likely to die, than patients with healthy body weight.[52-55]

The new strategy recognizes that 'tackling obesity is not just about an individual's effort, it is also about ... the choices that we are offered; and the influences that shape those choices.' It signals stronger intent to use legislation in place of voluntary mechanisms—including obligatory calorie labelling in restaurants and cafes; plus a ban on TV advertising to children of foods high in sugar or salt. As of December 2020, its implementation and effects remain to be seen.

Relieving the burden of choice

This comparison of tobacco and sugar offers a series of general lessons for alleviating 'behavioural' risks in the prevention of chronic and fatal diseases.

Prices affect supply and demand, for sugar and tobacco as for other commodities. Taxes, when carefully designed and calibrated, are a powerful way to reduce consumption, provided there is a collective will to apply them. Taxes bring the future into the present, presenting consumers and manufacturers with choices. Consumers can pay a price today for the costs incurred to themselves and to society in future, or save the money, adopt healthier lifestyles now, and avoid the later costs. Manufacturers, if faced with reduced demand (e.g. for tobacco or sugar), might choose to reduce production.

However, taxation works for citizens and government because it is only partially effective in changing unhealthy behaviour. Tax revenues depend on a sub-population of resolute consumers whose demand is resistant (inelastic) to price increases.[55] If everyone gave up smoking, there would be no income from tobacco sales. In practice, higher taxes on sugar and tobacco tend to reduce consumption by less than the increase in price, so taxation generally does raise revenue for governments.[3] People on lower incomes, who generally suffer more ill health due to sugar and tobacco, tend to be more responsive to price increases than wealthier people: they need and want help to improve their health and well-being, and they gain disproportionately.

If taxes benefit governments and consumers, why are they under-used?[56] In 2018, only 10% of the world's population were living in countries where cigarette taxes were 75% or more of the retail price, the minimum recommended by WHO.[19] The same problem applies to sugar and carbon (Chapter 8). There are three main reasons.

First, efficiency. Tax systems are not always easy to design and implement, but there are some general rules: taxes should be easy to administer, hard to manipulate, and difficult to game; they should employ simple mechanisms, such as uniform taxes on specific goods.[3]

Second, trust. Taxes are less acceptable to consumers when governments are not trusted to reinvest the revenue for public benefit. Tobacco-tax revenues currently add up to $270 billion per year globally, but less than $1 billion of that is spent on anti-smoking policies. Trust is built on diverse experiences, ranging from the shared success of co-production (cf. sanitation in Brazil; Chapter 7) to the shared identity of a cultural or tribal group (HIV/AIDS in Botswana; Chapter 5).[7,57,58]

Third, conflicts of interest. The sugar and tobacco industries will defend their commercial interests by means that are more and less legitimate.[59] Awareness is the basis of counter-defence: subversive industry tactics include lobbying and litigating against sugar and tobacco control policies, businesses colluding to counter government control efforts, and industries circumventing or disobeying laws and misrepresenting scientific evidence.[19]

Legislation is usually needed to align the interests of private businesses with the goals of public health; voluntary codes of conduct are mostly ineffective.[60,61] Clear statements of fact about taxation are required to counter industry misinformation (cf. the COVID-19 'infodemic', Chapter 4). Some of the relevant facts are: Taxes do not cause significant job losses in manufacturing industries because consumers usually buy other goods and services instead, shifting jobs from one sector to another sector. Higher taxes do not encourage tax avoidance or illicit trade. And increases in tobacco and food taxes have consistently produced revenues plus health benefits,[3] although the revenues are often the dominant force.[62]

Preventing illness and promoting health

Preventing illness (averting losses) and promoting good health (making gains) should be complementary.

Diet and exercise are two examples. Like taxes on unhealthy foods, subsidies that cut the cost of healthy foods encourage better food choices, provided the price reductions are large enough (10%–15%).[63]

Strong incentives are also needed to combat physical inactivity, a leading cause of mortality worldwide.[64,65] Although sedentary populations are notoriously immovable,[66] there are notable successes. Parkrun is a 5-km weekend run launched in the UK in 2004, which now takes place at around 1,400 locations in 22 countries worldwide.[67,68] Organized by volunteers, it has been successful in getting people active, probably because it offers a variety of benefits, which offset the comparatively low cost and effort of joining in. Parkrun is a means of health promotion but it is as much a social as a sporting event. Group running satisfies a range of motivations, from weight loss to speed gain, from getting out into the park to meeting friends at the weekend. There are strict but simple rules, which are applied everywhere, from Siberia to Soweto to San Francisco; and even in prisons in Australia, Ireland, and the UK. There is no need to be a hard-core runner; almost anyone can complete the short course—running, jogging, or walking. Parkrun is free to enter, takes place in the open air and under natural light, and is not tied to an indoor gym subscription. There is no upper time limit, no upper age limit, and there is no need for special equipment. Parkrun is sociable but also personal: each participant gets a time for the course, or a record of volunteering. They can use their own data to set benchmarks for improvement and compare their performances with friends and competitors. But only if they want to.

Summary

Consumers are ultimately responsible for 'behavioural' risks to their health, but the behaviours in question are also those of manufacturers and governments, and the burden of choice on consumers is lighter when shared. Governments, in particular, have the motives, means, and powers to intervene between commercial supply and consumer demand. Among the most effective instruments of government are taxation and regulation, especially for the control of single, major causes of illness such as tobacco and sugar. Taxes put a value on the future, today: consumers and manufacturers can choose to pay immediately for the costs incurred to society in future, or switch to healthier lifestyles and business practices. In practice, governments under pressure from lobbyists tend to under-tax harmful commodities, so other enticements are needed too. In this context, empirical studies show that health promotion is complementary to disease prevention—making health gains while avoiding health losses—especially when the joint benefits for health are large.

References

1. Lawton G. *This Book Could Save Your Life: The Science of Living Longer Better*. London: New Scientist; 2020.
2. James Baldwin. *No Name in the Street*. Penguin Random House; 1972.
3. The Task Force on Fiscal Policy for Health. *Health Taxes to Save Lives: Employing Effective Excise Taxes on Tobacco, Alcohol, and Sugary Beverages*. New York: Bloomberg Philanthropies; 2019.

4. Smith A. *An Inquiry into the Nature and Causes of the Wealth of Nations*. London: W. Strahan and T. Cadell; 1776.

5. Department of Health and Social Care. *Prevention Is Better than Cure: Our Vision to Help You Live Well for Longer*. London: Department of Health and Social Care; 2018.

6. Campbell D. People must take responsibility for own health, says Matt Hancock. 2018. https://www.theguardian.com/society/2018/nov/05/people-must-take-responsibility-for-own-health-says-matt-hancock (accessed 7 January 2021).

7. Wanless D. *Securing Good Health for the Whole Population*. London: Her Majesty's Stationery Office; 2004.

8. Institute for Health Metrics and Evaluation (IHME). GBD Results Tool. 2020. http://ghdx.healthdata.org/gbd-results-tool (accessed 7 January 2021).

9. GBD Risk Factors Collaborators. Global burden of 87 risk factors in 204 countries and territories, 1990–2019: A systematic analysis for the Global Burden of Disease Study 2019. *Lancet* 2020; *396*: 1223–49.

10. National Statistics (Information Services Division). *Cancer Incidence and Prevalence in Scotland (to December 2017)*. Edinburgh: National Statistics (Information Services Division); 2019.

11. National Statistics (Information Services Division). *Cancer Mortality in Scotland (2017)*. Edinburgh: National Statistics (Information Services Division); 2019.

12. World Health Organization. *WHO Global Report on Trends in Prevalence of Tobacco Use 2000–2025*. Geneva: World Health Organization; 2019.

13. Jha P, Peto R. Global effects of smoking, of quitting, and of taxing tobacco. *New England Journal of Medicine* 2014; *370*: 60–8.

14. World Health Organization. *WHO Global Report on Trends in Prevalence of Tobacco Smoking 2000–2025*. Geneva: World Health Organization; 2018.

15. Yeh CY, Schafferer C, Lee JM, Ho LM, Hsieh CJ. The effects of a rise in cigarette price on cigarette consumption, tobacco taxation revenues, and of smoking-related deaths in 28 EU countries—Applying threshold regression modelling. *BMC Public Health* 2017; *17*: 676.

16. Banks E, Joshy G, Weber MF, et al. Tobacco smoking and all-cause mortality in a large Australian cohort study: Findings from a mature epidemic with current low smoking prevalence. *BMC Medicine* 2015; *13*: 38.

17. Chesson H, Viscusi WK. The heterogeneity of time-risk tradeoffs. *Journal of Behavioral Decision Making* 2000; *13*: 251–8.

18. Peretti-Watel P, Seror V, Verger P, Guignard R, Legleye S, Beck F. Smokers' risk perception, socioeconomic status and source of information on cancer. *Addictive Behaviors* 2014; *39*: 1304–10.

19. Drope J, Schluger N, Cahn Z, et al. *The Tobacco Atlas*. Atlanta: American Cancer Society and Vital Strategies; 2018.

20. Hiscock R, Dobbie F, Bauld L. Smoking cessation and socioeconomic status: An update of existing evidence from a national evaluation of English stop smoking services. *BioMed Research International*, 2015; *2015*: 274056.

21. Hiscock R, Bauld L, Amos A, Platt S. Smoking and socioeconomic status in England: The rise of the never smoker and the disadvantaged smoker. *Journal of Public Health (Oxford)* 2012; *34*: 390–6.

22. Casetta B, Videla AJ, Bardach AP, et al. Association between cigarette smoking prevalence and income level: A systematic review and meta-analysis. *Nicotine & Tobacco Research* 2017: 1401–7.

23. Centers for Disease Control and Prevention. Smoking cessation: Fast facts. 2020. https://www.cdc.gov/tobacco/data_statistics/fact_sheets/fast_facts/index.htm#cigarette-smoking (accessed 7 January 2021).

24. World Health Organization. Tobacco. 2020. https://www.who.int/news-room/fact-sheets/detail/tobacco (accessed 7 January 2021).

25. Schmidt H, Gostin LO, Emanuel EJ. Public health, universal health coverage, and Sustainable Development Goals: Can they coexist? *Lancet* 2015; *386*: 928–30.

26. Levy DT, Yuan Z, Luo Y, Mays D. Seven years of progress in tobacco control: An evaluation of the effect of nations meeting the highest level MPOWER measures between 2007 and 2014. *Tobacco Control* 2018; *27*: 50–7.

27. Sugar TaATG. Sugar, tobacco, and alcohol taxes to achieve the SDGs. *Lancet* 2018; *391*: 2400–1.

28. Whitehead R, Brown L, Riches E, et al. *Strengths and Limitations of Tobacco Taxation and Pricing Strategies.* Edinburgh: NHS Health Scotland; 2018.

29. The Cancer Council. Price elasticity of demand for tobacco products. 2019. https://www.tobaccoinaustralia.org.au/home.aspx.

30. Goodchild M, Perucic AM, Nargis N. Modelling the impact of raising tobacco taxes on public health and finance. *Bulletin of the World Health Organization* 2016; *94*: 250–7.

31. Jha P, MacLennan M, Chaloupka FJ, et al. Global hazards of tobacco and the benefits of smoking cessation and tobacco taxes. In: Gelband H, Jha P, Sankaranarayanan R, Horton S, eds. *Cancer Disease Control Priorities.* 3rd edn. Washington, DC: World Bank; 2015: 175–93.

32. The Economist. How to cut smoking in poor countries. The Economist. 1 June 2017.

33. Centers for Disease Control and Prevention. Within 20 minutes of quitting poster. 2004. https://www.cdc.gov/tobacco/data_statistics/sgr/2004/posters/20mins/index.htm (accessed 7 January 2021).

34. Cleave TL. *The Saccharine Disease.* Bristol: John Wright & Sons Limited; 1974.

35. Te Morenga L, Mallard S, Mann J. Dietary sugars and body weight: Systematic review and meta-analyses of randomised controlled trials and cohort studies. *BMJ* 2012; *345*: e7492.

36. Guh DP, Zhang W, Bansback N, Amarsi Z, Birmingham CL, Anis AH. The incidence of co-morbidities related to obesity and overweight: A systematic review and meta-analysis. *BMC Public Health* 2009; *9*: 88.

37. Akbaraly TN, Brunner EJ, Ferrie JE, Marmot MG, Kivimaki M, Singh-Manoux A. Dietary pattern and depressive symptoms in middle age. *British Journal of Psychiatry* 2009; *195*: 408–13.

38. Yang Q, Zhang Z, Gregg EW, Flanders WD, Merritt R, Hu FB. Added sugar intake and cardiovascular diseases mortality among US adults. *JAMA Internal Medicine* 2014; *174*: 516–24.
39. Speakman JR. Evolutionary perspectives on the obesity epidemic: Adaptive, maladaptive, and neutral viewpoints. *Annual Review of Nutrition* 2013; *33*: 289–317.
40. Uusitupa M, Lindstrom J, Tuomilehto J. Prevention of type 2 diabetes—success story that is waiting for next steps. *European Journal of Clinical Nutrition* 2018; *72*: 1260–6.
41. von Philipsborn P, Stratil JM, Burns J, et al. Environmental interventions to reduce the consumption of sugar-sweetened beverages and their effects on health. *Cochrane Database of Systematic Reviews* 2019; *6*: CD012292.
42. Backholer K, Vandevijvere S, Blake M, Tseng M. Sugar-sweetened beverage taxes in 2018: A year of reflections and consolidation. *Public Health Nutrition* 2018; *21*: 3291–5.
43. Grummon AH, Lockwood BB, Taubinsky D, Allcott H. Designing better sugary drink taxes. *Science* 2019; *365*: 989–90.
44. Hashem KM, He FJ, MacGregor GA. Labelling changes in response to a tax on sugar-sweetened beverages, United Kingdom of Great Britain and Northern Ireland. *Bulletin of the World Health Organization* 2019; *97*: 818–27.
45. Scarborough P, Adhikari V, Harrington RA, Elhussein A, Briggs A, Rayner M, et al. Impact of the announcement and implementation of the UK Soft Drinks Industry Levy on sugar content, price, product size and number of available soft drinks in the UK, 2015-19: A controlled interrupted time series analysis. *PLoS Medicine* 2020; *17*: e1003025.
46. Bandy LK, Scarborough P, Harrington RA, Rayner M, Jebb SA. Reductions in sugar sales from soft drinks in the UK from 2015 to 2018. *BMC Medicine* 2020; *18*: 20.
47. Obesity Evidence Hub. Countries that have implemented taxes on sugar-sweetened beverages (SSBs). https://www.obesityevidencehub.org.au/collections/prevention/countries-that-have-implemented-taxes-on-sugar-sweetened-beverages-ssbs (accessed 7 January 2021).
48. Arthur R, Watson E, Michail N, Scattergood G, Southey F. Sugar taxes: The global picture. 2019. https://www.foodnavigator-latam.com/Article/2019/12/18/Sugar-taxes-The-global-picture-in-2019 (accessed 7 January 2021).
49. Scheelbeek PFD, Cornelsen L, Marteau TM, Jebb SA, Smith RD. Potential impact on prevalence of obesity in the UK of a 20% price increase in high sugar snacks: Modelling study. *BMJ* 2019; *366*: l4786.
50. Public Health England. *Sugar Reduction: Report on Progress between 2015 and 2018*. London: Public Health England; 2019.
51. National Audit Office. *Childhood Obesity*. London: National Audit Office; 2020.
52. Department of Health and Social Care. Tackling obesity: Empowering adults and children to live healthier lives. 2020. https://www.gov.uk/government/publications/tackling-obesity-government-strategy/tackling-obesity-empowering-adults-and-children-to-live-healthier-lives (accessed 7 January 2021).

53. Public Health England. *Excess Weight and COVID-19: Insights from New Evidence*. London: Public Health England; 2020.
54. Popkin BM, Du S, Green WD, et al. Individuals with obesity and COVID-19: A global perspective on the epidemiology and biological relationships. *Obesity Reviews* 2020; *21*: e13128.
55. Liu F. Sin taxes: Have governments gone too far in their efforts to monetize morality? *Boston College Law Review* 2018; *59*: 763–89.
56. Gostin LO, Monahan JT, Kaldor J, et al. The legal determinants of health: Harnessing the power of law for global health and sustainable development. *Lancet* 2019; *393*: 1857–910.
57. Acemoglu D, Robinson JA. *Why Nations Fail: The Origins of Power, Prosperity and Poverty*. New York: Crown Publishing Group; 2012.
58. Ostrom E, *Governing the Commons: The Evolution of Institutions for Collective Action*. New York: Cambridge University Press; 1990.
59. Eykelenboom M, van Stralen MM, Olthof MR, et al. Political and public acceptability of a sugar-sweetened beverages tax: A mixed-method systematic review and meta-analysis. *International Journal of Behavioral Nutrition and Physical Activity* 2019; *16*: 78.
60. Powell L. Progress in reducing food sugar content 'lost' as people buying more, Public Health England warns. The Independent. 29 October 2019.
61. Kaldor JC, Thow AM, Schönfeldt H. Using regulation to limit salt intake and prevent non-communicable diseases: Lessons from South Africa's experience. *Public Health Nutrition* 2019; *22*: 1316–25.
62. Jensen JD, Smed S. State-of-the-art for food taxes to promote public health. *Proceedings of the Nutrition Society* 2018; *77*: 100–5.
63. Niebylski ML, Redburn KA, Duhaney T, Campbell NR. Healthy food subsidies and unhealthy food taxation: A systematic review of the evidence. *Nutrition* 2015; *31*: 787–95.
64. World Health Organization. *Global Health Risks: Mortality and Burden of Disease Attributable to Selected Major Risks*. Geneva: World Health Organization; 2009.
65. World Health Organization. *Global Recommendations on Physical Activity for Health*. Geneva: World Health Organization; 2010.
66. Pratt M, Ramirez Varela A, Salvo D, Kohl Iii HW, Ding D. Attacking the pandemic of physical inactivity: What is holding us back? *British Journal of Sports Medicine* 2020; *54*: 760–2.
67. Parkrun. 2020. https://www.parkrun.com/ (accessed 8 September 2020).
68. Reece LJ, Quirk H, Wellington C, Haake SJ, Wilson F. Bright Spots, physical activity investments that work: Parkrun; a global initiative striving for healthier and happier communities. *British Journal of Sports Medicine* 2019; *53*: 326–7.

7
The culture of conveniences

Water is life, sanitation is dignity.
UK Department for International Development (2007)[1]

Water and life trump sanitation and dignity, with major consequences for health. Despite thousands of years of toilet culture and technology, the great majority of people alive today do not have access to safe sanitation. The challenge of sanitation as a means of prevention is to align the benefits to health with personal and social preferences for toilet use and hygiene, while exploiting other advantages for agriculture, energy, education, environmental protection, housing, and flood protection. To get the most out of sanitation requires cooperation among many kinds of providers and users—individuals, communities, businesses, financial donors, and governments—who have different needs in different settings. To make a compelling case for investment in sanitation, economic evaluations should go further than conventional cost-benefit analyses, which typically ignore the cultural constraints and neglect most of the social benefits.

The bottom four billion

A 2007 survey for a top medical journal voted sanitation the greatest medical advance since 1840—ahead of antibiotics, anaesthesia, and vaccines—even though health was just one of sanitation's many benefits (Chapters 1 and 2).[2] The enormous value of sanitation, for the health of individuals, families, and communities, has been understood for millennia (Chapter 1). And yet the state of the world's toilets and sewers today is parlous. Every country has signed up to the goal of achieving safe sanitation for all by 2030, in line with the Sustainable Development Goals (SDGs), but few will reach that target. In 2017, more than four billion people (55% of the world

The Great Health Dilemma. Christopher Dye, Oxford University Press. © Oxford University Press 2021.
DOI: 10.1093/oso/9780198853824.003.0007

population) did not have access to a 'safely managed'[3] sanitary system that prevents exposure to excreta; two billion (27%) did not live in a household with any kind of toilet; and around 900 million people still practised open defecation.[4,5] At the same time, the world's most fortunate people—the top billion—had the luxury of defecating into water that was almost clean enough to drink.

The proportion of people worldwide with access to at least 'basic sanitation' (facilities that are not shared with other households)[3] increased by less than one percentage point per year between 2000 and 2017 (from 59% to 68%), and coverage was well below the global average in low-income countries (Figure 7.1). A larger fraction of the world's population was 'open defecation free' in 2017, but only 18 of 62 countries were on track to eliminate open defecation by 2030; in eight countries, the proportion of people openly defecating actually increased between 2000 and 2017.

There is a large gap between ending open defecation and acquiring basic sanitation (Figure 7.1). That exists because 'basic sanitation' refers to facilities that are not shared with other households. Community toilets could

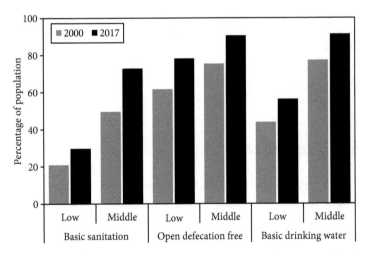

Figure 7.1 Trends in water and sanitation. Changes in the coverage of basic sanitation, basic drinking water, and the elimination of open defecation in low- and middle-income countries between 2000 and 2017. The elimination of open defecation and the coverage of basic drinking water are farther advanced than basic sanitation.

Source: Data from World Bank. World Bank Open Data. 2019. https://data.worldbank.org/

help bridge the gap, as they have for example in Mumbai, India (below).[6] But shared toilets need shared ownership if they are to remain safe, comfortable, and hygienic.

Comparing progress in the provision of drinking water (faster) and sanitation (slower) points to the effects of different incentives (Figure 7.1). Although drinking and defecating are both necessities, a safe water supply is needed every day but safe sanitation is not. Water typically comes from a central source (spring, well, river) that must be cooperatively managed, whereas there are multiple sites to defecate in the environment. Open defecation is not only possible, particularly in rural areas of Africa and Asia, but also socially acceptable. Public willingness to pay for sanitation and wastewater treatment is consequently lower than for the provision of drinking water, and unit costs are usually higher.[7] Water is talked about openly, in terms of water purity, well-being, and quality of life, and attracts public champions; defecation, like other private bodily functions, draws imaginative euphemisms and few public advocates.[8] Sanitation also commonly loses out to water when setting policy and budgetary priorities, particularly when controlled by water ministries.[1]

The slow progress in sanitation is at odds with numerous economic evaluations that conclude that sanitation is good value for money. A 2012 World Health Organization (WHO) study calculated that every US dollar invested in sanitation would deliver a return of US$5.50 (range US$2.8–8.0 across nine regions of the world) in lower health costs, fewer premature deaths, and greater economic productivity.[10–14] Such favourable rewards are intended to encourage investment by governments and international donors but, judged by the slow progress, they have been less persuasive than expected. There are broadly two possible reasons: the costs of safe sanitation are too high; or the benefits are too low. Both costs and benefits should be broadly defined—beyond money.

First, the costs. Estimates of the money needed are large—much larger than the funds currently available—which raises the question of whether safe sanitation is affordable, and on what timescale. Current global levels of financing are sufficient to cover only the capital costs of achieving basic sanitation (as part of WASH [water, sanitation, and hygiene]) by 2030, and provided funds are directed to the people who are in greatest need (based on Trackfin, Chapter 2).[15,16] Governments presently contribute only a fifth of all funding for WASH; two-thirds comes from households. Meeting SDG targets for 'safely managed' water and sanitation (the higher, health-safe standard) will require a tripling of capital investments to US$114 billion per year, to which must be added the operations and maintenance (O&M) costs that are vital for service continuity.[15] After initial capital expenditure, O&M costs will make up an increasing fraction of WASH budgets, and place a significant financial burden on the poorest households. The present funding gap is therefore huge, and safe sanitation may demand much more than governments and households are willing or able to afford.

Second, the benefits. The WHO study calculated the major economic value of sanitation to be in time savings (81%), augmented by lower healthcare costs (8%), and greater longevity (6%) and labour productivity (5%).[12] But many other potential benefits were excluded, as the authors made clear: for agriculture (nutrients for soil fertility), energy (excreta recycled for fuel), education (school attendance), environment (water reuse, safety, and security), housing (sanitary assets), infrastructure (access roads, flood protection), and quality of life (personal safety, convenience, dignity, gender equality).[12] All these assets, if they can be acquired, suggest that the potential benefits of sanitation have been undervalued. Sanitation could therefore yield substantially more than the calculated fivefold (average) return, depending on the technology (pit latrines, septic tanks), making it still more competitive as an investment for development (with the usual caveats on benefit/cost ratios; Box 2.1).[12,17]

There are, however, important qualifications to the idea that sanitation can deliver large benefits if only the costs are affordable. One of these is that the perceived costs, benefits, and minimum requirements for sanitation, which govern choice, differ among individuals, communities, businesses, donors, and governments, all of whom have the power to influence decisions. Unless sanitation is valued by all those who have a stake, it is not likely to succeed. The true return on investment could, in practice, be anything from enormous to negligible, depending on the degree of cooperation.

With that background, the rest of the chapter considers the value of sanitation to all stakeholders: with respect to individual and population health, including the prevention of epidemics; in satisfying personal preferences and social norms for toilet use and hygienic behaviour; in gaining strength from cooperation, locally and nationally; and in contributing to sustainable development.

Dialogue on Diarrhoea

The idea of sanitation is rooted in health and hygiene, but the value of sanitation for health is likely to differ from the perspective of individuals and populations. The *Dialogue on Diarrhoea* was an international newsletter, published by the non-governmental organization (NGO) Healthlink Worldwide from 1980 to 1995, to discuss all aspects of the control of diarrhoeal diseases.

Health-safe sanitation prevents exposure to faeces, mainly the faeces of other people or animals, which are sources of new infections with an array of disease-causing pathogens (Chapter 2).[18] Among them are bacteria—*Vibrio cholerae* (cholera), *Cryptosporidium*, *Shigella* (dysentery), enterotoxigenic *Escherichia coli* (*E. coli* is also a marker of environmental contamination with faeces), *Salmonella* (typhoid), and *Chlamydia* (blinding trachoma), some of them now resistant to antibiotics. There are viruses—adenovirus (conjunctivitis), polio, hepatitis A, and rotavirus; parasites—*Necator* and *Ancylostoma* (hookworms), *Ascaris* (roundworm), and *Schistosoma* (bilharzia); and fungi such as *Tinea* (ringworm). Open drains and sewers also provide breeding sites for the mosquito vectors of *Wuchereria* (filarial worms), *Plasmodium* (malaria), and West Nile virus, among others. As well as causing specific illnesses, infections contribute to, and are predisposed by, various forms of under-nutrition (stunting, wasting, vitamin and mineral deficiencies), losing school time for children, cutting the productivity of working adults, and shortening life expectancy.[19,20]

Given this parasitic onslaught, unsafe sanitation makes a large contribution to the avoidable burden of disease on populations. Each year, about 800,000 people in low- and middle-income countries die as a result of inadequate water, sanitation, or hygiene. Poor sanitation is the main cause of about 400,000 deaths due to diarrhoeal diseases. Clean water, safe sanitation, and hygiene could prevent the deaths of 300,000 children under 5 years old annually, with the positive returns on investment reported above.[4]

But for sanitation to succeed, supply (from providers) must meet demand (from users). Although the risk of infection from unsafe sanitation is persistently high in many low-income countries, the risk of a severe or fatal outcome is small. Even in South Asia and Sub-Saharan Africa, where children under 5 years old typically suffer two to three episodes of diarrhoea each year, most episodes are mild and self-resolving; fewer than 2 in 100 are severe and case fatality rarely exceeds 2 in a 1,000.[21,22] In these settings, childhood diarrhoea is sometimes viewed as a chronic normal, an accepted and low-value part of everyday life, albeit with occasional outbreaks of severe disease such as cholera (below).

If individual people (low disease risk) and public health authorities (high disease burden) attach different values to sanitation, and are also presented with different costs, these differences may need to be reconciled to encourage collaboration.

Both individuals and public health authorities are also usually aware that there are alternative methods of prevention (vaccines) and cheap and effective treatments for diarrhoea (oral rehydration therapy). In principle, these are disincentives for prevention through sanitation.

Sanitation in the time of cholera

John Snow's famous investigation of cholera has forever linked the disease with a failure to provide clean water and safe sanitation. But although cholera was greatly feared in London and other cities during the nineteenth century, it was only one motive, albeit a prominent one, for sanitary reform. There were many more deaths routinely from other endemic infections. The need to remove human waste was a powerful factor too: the stink of faeces took cesspits out of houses, and the stink of the Thames led to the removal of faeces from the river (Chapter 1).

Cholera outbreaks today are still commonplace in Africa, Asia, and the Americas and remain 'potentially notifiable events' under International Health Regulations (IHR) 2005 (Chapter 4), but they are nowadays usually local rather than national or international emergencies. They make a small contribution to the number of deaths from diarrhoeal diseases, but attract disproportionate attention and remain a signal of need for safe sanitation.[23] That need is not easily satisfied during an outbreak, when long-term solutions are side-lined in favour of short-term emergency responses—including the provision of clean water for drinking and washing, targeted vaccination to contain an outbreak, and reactive treatment to prevent severe illness and death.

The benefits of preventing a severe outbreak of disease linked to unsafe sanitation—whether it be cholera, dysentery, or typhoid—must be carried over to 'peace time' and added to sanitation's other benefits. One way to bridge the gap is by linking short- and long-term responses—for example, by tying the provision of cholera vaccines, not just to immediate solutions (water treatment and storage, provision of soap, promotion of handwashing), but also to systematic analyses of need for long-term investment in sanitation.[24]

Preferences and prohibitions

The poorest people in society are not just penniless: they are also relatively powerless. But they do sometimes have the power of refusal. Toilets can only contribute to safe sanitation if people are willing to use them.

For individuals, families, communities, and schools, toilets are not merely, or even mainly, for health. People are primarily concerned about whether toilets are available, accessible, and acceptable,[1,3] rather than with the management of excreta as a health hazard. Acceptability hinges on convenience, privacy, safety, and dignity, where personal preferences are rooted in cultural beliefs and social norms.[1,25,26]

Some of the reasons why people do not use toilets are obvious—because they are broken, blocked, dirty, or overflowing—and the technical solutions are obvious too. Less easy to understand and modify are long-standing sanitary behaviours based on local customs. Abundant research studies have shown how sanitary preferences are expressed in different settings: in Eastern Zambia, male heads of household prefer not to share toilets with women and children when there is a high risk of being seen.[27] In Bangladesh, men avoid sharing toilets with women to prevent mutual embarrassment during menstruation, preferring instead to defecate outdoors.[28]

In India, Hindu beliefs about purity and pollution mean that open defecation is personally preferable and socially acceptable. Open defecation is not a hardship to be overcome: it is believed to be good for health, pleasurable, wholesome, comfortable, and convenient.[29-31] Toilets, on the other hand, are thought to pollute the environment in and around dwellings.[27,30] Open defecation is gradually disappearing (Figure 7.1) but the transition to toilet use is not irreversible.[32] In rural Laos, for example, some households unable to pay US$50 to empty a latrine have reverted to open defecation.[27]

In rural India, some government-provided, low-cost ('affordable') pit latrines are unused by Hindus because they have to be emptied manually—degrading work that is traditionally done by dalits or 'untouchables' (Figure 7.2). Rural Hindus prefer more costly latrines, if they can afford them, which can be emptied by machine or which need not be emptied at all, or they defecate in the open.[29] Up-market latrines with large pits or cemented

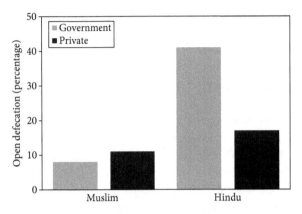

Figure 7.2 Open defecation in Muslim and Hindu communities of India. Percentage of people who live in households with latrines but practise open defecation, by religion and type of latrine (government-provided or private), in five states. Private latrines are typically large pits or cemented underground tanks, which are perceived to be non-polluting and more desirable. The government provides simple soak pits, which are smaller and less acceptable, especially for Hindus.

Adapted with permission from Coffey, D., Gupta, A., Hathi, P., *et al.* (2017). Understanding open defecation in rural India. Untouchability, pollution, and latrine pits. *Economic & Political Weekly*; 52: 59–66.

underground tanks are seen as household assets whereas latrines with small soak pits, such as those provided by the government, are often unused.[29] Indian Muslims, in contrast, are more likely to use the latrines that they own, whether private or provided by the government, and fewer defecate openly (Figure 7.2). In Muslim Bangladesh, a combination of approaches—subsidies, micro-credit, improved sanitation markets, and others—means that the majority of households now use latrines, and open defecation has essentially been eliminated.[28,33]

Sub-standard sanitation presents special problems for women and girls. A lack of suitable facilities during menstruation means that girls miss days at school or college. Poor-quality toilets, and shared toilets, leave women vulnerable to violence.[28,34,35] In some settings without household toilets, women must defecate outdoors before dawn, or hold out until after dark.

These are some of the factors that determine the value of toilets and sanitation, and therefore the choices made by individuals and communities. They explain why simply providing a toilet, even if cheap and functional, does not guarantee that it will be used.[1] The difficulty of judging which of many factors are important in any particular setting may also explain why standard information, education, and communication ('total sanitation') campaigns struggle to improve health by changing sanitary behaviour.[36,37]

Personal preferences are shaped by social norms and their observance is a form of cooperation. But sanitation demands other forms of cooperation too, including a consensus on the needs of a community of users with respect to offers from public and private providers. Some examples follow.

Bottom up meets top down

Sanitary improvements made by individuals have limited benefits, both for those individuals and for whole communities. Leaky latrines contaminate the environmental commons, and pit latrines cannot easily be integrated into communal sewage systems. To maximize its social and cultural value, and its benefits for health, sanitation needs cooperation.

Community participation is one of the 'means of implementation' of SDG 6 but, as for other SDGs, little guidance is given on what the means should be.[5] Clearly, there is a need for dialogue, which can take many forms, such as WASH committees at village level (e.g. Laos, Rwanda, Tanzania, and Zimbabwe) or in workshops to develop national WASH policies and strategies (Costa Rica, Senegal).[5]

The purpose of the dialogue is to understand preferences and resolve differences. In six villages in rural Tanzania, the technologies that users found to be socially and economically acceptable (e.g. an improved floor toilet with a washable cement surface) were different from those recommended by sanitation experts (e.g. prefabricated concrete platforms, constructed by skilled artisans), and opinions differed among villages.[38] Among rural Quilombola communities in Brazil, dry systems were recommended by experts to reduce water consumption, but rejected by communities more comfortable with flushing toilets. Given local preferences for flushing toilets, for recycling water, and to create an environment attractive to tourists, the community opted for a system of evapotranspiration of blackwater (zero discharge from toilets), with greywater (from cooking and washing) used to irrigate banana tree gardens.[39]

The demand for toilets and other sanitary products, and for removing human waste, is met by private as well as public suppliers worldwide.[1] Small-scale, private providers have been vital to the success of community-led total sanitation (CLTS) programmes, which originated in Bangladesh. The goal of CLTS is to eliminate open defecation, offering instead subsidized construction of toilets, household by household.[22] Motivating people through social pressure (mixing reward and shame), CLTS has been a powerful, if controversial, tool for social mobilization.[40,41]

A key feature of CLTS has been the design and construction of latrines to a price rather than to a specification; capped prices make toilets affordable for poorer people. Another is the way in which potentially conflicting opinions have been resolved at community level, putting, for example, individual rights to privacy and dignity alongside social and economic entitlements to sanitation.[41] In general, the assertion that sanitation is a human right[42] rarely has force unless accompanied by practical instruments that influence choices—such as laws, regulations, and ethical codes that deliver tangible benefits such as finance, training, and technology.

The Orangi Pilot Project (OPP), which began in 1980 in Karachi's largest slum,[6] has become a well-known story of communal action driven by the demand for sanitation.[43] But OPP also illustrates the difficulty of aligning interests, of creating a replicable model, and of expanding it nationally. Community social innovation, linked to appropriate technology (simple sewers), generated a low-cost sanitation system. Orangi residents were given technical and organizational support to build a sanitary latrine in each house, an underground sewer in each 'lane' (20–40 households), and a collector sewer in each neighbourhood, the latter feeding into a trunk sewer provided by the government. Gordon McGranahan and Diana Mitlin explain the importance of cooperation that makes connections from households to cities:

> If the state did not provide the trunk sewer, the collector sewer would pollute the city, if the neighbourhood did not provide the collector sewer the lane sewer would pollute the neighbourhood, and if the lane did not provide their sewer the household's sewage would pollute the lane.

To borrow an Indian metaphor, it is not a question of dividing responsibility for 'big pipes' (government) and 'little pipes' (households);[6] rather, it is a question of sharing responsibility because neither big pipes nor little pipes are useful unless joined together.[44,45]

Connecting pipes is symbolic of what Elinor Ostrom and her collaborators called 'co-production', when bottom up meets top down: providers and consumers, government planners and citizens, collaborate to make sanitation (in this case) work, and to reduce costs. Their example, in north-east Brazil, showed how condominial sewers, serving housing blocks inhabited by people on low incomes, were an affordable and effective sanitation system, provided local planners and contractors were willing to work with residents.[18,46] Condominial sewer pipes are smaller than conventional pipes and laid closer to the surface, and they are less than half the price of a conventional sewage system. Coproduction worked in north-east Brazil because residents co-designed the layout, making their own choices between cheaper and more costly options and, on the basis of agreement, committing to pay a fee.

The mechanism of coproduction depends on context. The Indian Alliance of NGOs was created in Mumbai in the 1980s, primarily to secure permanent housing for women pavement dwellers. Sanitation has been central to their strategy.[6] Women who came together to create credit and savings groups, a source of small loans, were also able to look after community toilets. Public toilets are built for anyone and owned by no-one, whereas a community toilet is held jointly by a defined and responsible group of people. The improvements made to community toilets, incrementally and iteratively, contributed to the primary aim of upgrading houses, and in giving residents security of tenure.

These examples of custom-made solutions (social, technical, financial) for sanitation on small scales (households, city neighbourhoods, villages) point to the challenges of replicating successful projects in other settings and on larger scales (cities and countries).

A nation of communities

Planning from the top down only succeeds when it accommodates needs expressed from the bottom up—when supply satisfies demand. Nevertheless, national success in sanitation needs a national strategy, leadership, and a means of implementation (as it did in nineteenth-century Europe; Chapter 1).[47]

Malaysia, Singapore, Republic of Korea, and Thailand rapidly expanded the coverage of sanitation from the 1950s onwards. In each of these countries, strong leadership motivated by nation building came before increases in national wealth.[47] In the mould of nineteenth-century Europe (Chapter 1), national strategies for hygiene, cleanliness, and public health, coordinated across different sectors of government, drove improvements in sanitation (Health in All Policies; Chapter 3).

The integration of sanitation in the economic development of these four countries is more easily described than replicated, as revealed by the more recent but less successful outcomes in Pakistan, Philippines, and Bangladesh.

Based on the success in Karachi (above), the OPP approach to sanitation had been adopted by more than 90% of informal houses in Orangi by 2012—more than 100,000 households. But this is a long way from achieving safe sanitation nationwide.[43] In general, Pakistan has focused on eliminating open defecation rather than on the safe management of faecal waste, and there is extensive, continuing faecal contamination of surface and ground water. Untreated wastewater from houses is routinely used for crop irrigation, magnifying the risk of human infection and the contamination of food produce. As a result, the incidence of diarrhoeal disease is still high even among the wealthiest households in Karachi.[48]

In the Philippines, the Pasig River Rehabilitation Commission (PRRC) was created to clean up Manila's grossly polluted river system. Between 1999 and 2017, the PRRC resettled 18,000 families living along the riverbanks of one tributary of the river, dismantled 376 encroaching private structures, established environmental preservation areas along 37 kilometres of riverbanks, developed 17 of its 47 identified tributaries, diverted around 22 million kilograms of solid waste, and made this typhoon-prone area more resilient to flooding.[49] Although a celebrated case study in urban renewal, the PRRC also illustrates the problem of taking such an initiative beyond cooperative local communities to city scale. Oversight at the level of municipal Manila has failed: most of the Pasig River tributaries are still cesspools, the focus of regular complaints by the public and in the media.[50]

In Bangladesh, the 2003–06 national sanitation campaign based on CLTS was successful in combining top-down government and bottom-up community mobilization, and in shifting cultural norms so that open defecation became socially unacceptable in most parts of the country.[28] But there is a big gap between eliminating open defecation and achieving safe sanitation nationwide (Figure 7.1). Rural and urban environments are still extensively polluted with human and animal faeces. Many Bangladeshis have switched, not to modern sanitation facilities but to basic pit latrines shared with neighbours. Heavy use and uncertain ownership of these facilities compromise cleanliness, maintenance, and personal safety. And there remains a failure of cooperation in protecting people and the environment from harmful waste.[51]

These examples provide lessons on how to (and how not to) turn personal preferences into collective action, at small and large scales. They help map the route to universal safe sanitation in the age of sustainable development.

Sanitation and sustainable development

Between 1990 and 2015, sanitation was linked to all eight Millennium Development Goals (MDGs). The MDGs were conceived as a partnership between richer and poorer countries to end extreme poverty. Interventions targeted low-income countries with high burdens of disease and MDG 4 aimed to reduce the mortality rate of children under 5 years by two-thirds.[1,40] In the event, the child mortality rate was halved in low- and middle-income countries between 1990 and 2015, from 91 to 41 deaths per 1,000 live births (or 12.7 million to 5.9 million deaths/year). Although short of the target, that result counts as one of the great achievements of the MDG era. Success was attributed more to medical care (drugs supported by vaccination) than to prevention upstream, by means including WASH. Reflecting the MDG emphasis on treatment rather than prevention, the incidence of infection with diarrhoeal disease pathogens was largely un-diminished over 25 years.[22]

The unachieved MDGs (there were still 5.5 million mostly preventable deaths among children under 5 in 2017) have been carried over to, and ab-sorbed within, the SDGs (health goal SDG 3 includes target 3.2 on child mortality).[52,53] But the SDGs carry a far greater ambition than the MDGs—to anchor health in development, recognizing that good health depends on and contributes to other development goals, underpinning social justice, economic prosperity, and environmental protection. SDG 6 aims to 'ensure the availability and sustainable management of water and sanitation for all'.

SDG 6 contributes to, benefits from, or otherwise interacts with at least 12 of the other 16 SDGs (1–5, 8, 9, 11–15), including those concerned with poverty, nutrition, education, gender and other inequalities, economic growth, life in water and on land, and sustainable cities.[3,12,54–56] Specifically, householders can invest in sanitation as a property asset, especially if they are home owners rather than tenants.[6] The nutrients from excreta can be used as an agricultural fertilizer; solid waste can be converted to biofuel; wastewater can be recovered and purified or used for irrigation; sanitary engineering can help conserve water and prevent flooding; and sanitary structures (dykes, embankments, covered drains) can support access roads.[57] In the context of environmental protection, sanitation has a role in sustaining resource cycles—a 'nature-based solution' with potential benefits for whole ecosystems.[58,59] 'Regenerative sanitation' advocates resource recovery, reuse, and recycling, while 'ecological sanitation' aims to close nutrient and water cycles with minimal energy expenditure.[60,61] Among all these benefits are opportunities for business and tourism, which should be part of any comprehensive evaluation of the costs and benefits of sanitation. A snapshot of sanitation across the world today suggests that the transition from low to high coverage occurs mainly within the group of lower-middle income countries (Figure 7.3). Exceptions prove the rule: few low- or lower-middle income countries have population-wide sanitation coverage, but Rwanda and the former Soviet states Kyrgyz Republic and Tajikistan have unusually high coverage, given their wealth. Conversely, few wealthy countries have low sanitation coverage; Gabon and Namibia are, however, lagging behind other upper-middle income countries (Figure 7.3).

Malaysia, Singapore, Republic of Korea, and Thailand (upper-middle and high income) have shown how national sanitary systems are built

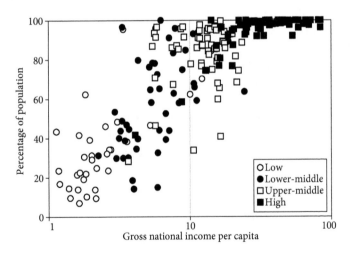

Figure 7.3 The sanitation transition. Association between sanitation and economic development: population coverage of 'basic sanitation' in countries grouped by gross national income (purchasing power parity, international $), 2015.

Source: Data from World Bank. World Bank Open Data. 2019. https://data.worldbank.org/

alongside efficient institutions and good governance, with legislation and regulations, skills and technology, monitoring and evaluation for transparency and accountability, and collaboration across departments and disciplines (Chapter 3).[15,16,47] Most people living in high-income countries today have access to hygienic household toilets with safe waste disposal; the creation of a safe sanitary system is one of the mutually reinforcing processes of social and economic development. This is as true in low- and lower-middle income countries today as it was in Europe during the nineteenth century (cf. Figure 1.1, Chapter 1).

Summary

Despite thousands of years of toilet culture and technology, and despite the obvious benefits of sanitation for health and well-being, the great majority of people alive today do not have access to a safe system for removing human waste. The installation of safe sanitary systems depends on cooperation among many kinds of providers and users. Their collective goal is to align the benefits for health with personal and social preferences for toilet use and hygiene, while exploiting other benefits from agriculture, energy, education, environmental protection, housing, and flood protection. For individuals, families, and communities, toilets are not merely, or even mainly, to protect health. Rather, their acceptability hinges on convenience, privacy, personal safety, and dignity, where preferences are rooted in societal norms. Providing safe sanitation for all is not merely a health intervention; it is one of the mutually reinforcing processes of cultural, social, and economic development.

References

1. Department for International Development (DFID) Sanitation Reference Group. *Sanitation Policy Background Paper. Water Is Life, Sanitation Is Dignity.* London: DFID; 2007.
2. Ferriman A. BMJ readers choose sanitation as greatest medical advance since 1840. *BMJ* 2007; *334*: 111.
3. World Health Organization. *Guidelines on Sanitation and Health.* Geneva: WHO; 2018.
4. United Nations Children's Fund (UNICEF) and World Health Organization. Progress on household drinking water, sanitation and hygiene 2000–2017: Special focus on inequalities. New York: UNICEF and WHO; 2019.

5. United Nations. *Sustainable Development Goal 6 Synthesis Report 2018 on Water and Sanitation*. New York: United Nations; 2018.

6. McGranahan G, Mitlin D. Learning from sustained success: How community-driven initiatives to improve urban sanitation can meet the challenges. *World Development* 2016; *87*: 307–17.

7. Bos JJ, Gijzen HJ, Hilderink HBM, Moussa M, Niessen LW, de Ruyter ED. Health benefits versus costs of water supply and sanitation. *Water* 2005; *7*: 1–6.

8. Editorial. We need to talk about crapping. *Nature Microbiology* 2018; *3*: 1189.

9. World Bank. World Bank open data. 2021. https://data.worldbank.org (accessed 7 January 2021).

10. World Health Organization. *Global Costs and Benefits of Drinking-Water Supply and Sanitation Interventions to Reach the MDG Target and Universal Coverage*. Geneva: WHO; 2012.

11. Hutton G, Chase C. The knowledge base for achieving the sustainable development goal targets on water supply, sanitation and hygiene. *International Journal of Environmental Research and Public Health* 2016; *13*: 536.

12. Hutton G. Global costs and benefits of reaching universal coverage of sanitation and drinking-water supply. *Journal of Water and Health* 2013; *11*: 1–12.

13. Hutton G, Haller L, Bartram J. Global cost-benefit analysis of water supply and sanitation interventions. *Journal of Water and Health* 2007; *5*: 481–502.

14. Hutton G, Chase C. Water supply, sanitation, and hygiene. In: Mock CN, Nugent R, Kobusingye O, Smith KR, eds. *Injury Prevention and Environmental Health*. Washington, DC: World Bank; 2017: 171–98.

15. Hutton G, Varughese MC. *The Costs of Meeting the 2030 Sustainable Development Goal Targets on Drinking Water, Sanitation, and Hygiene*. Washington, DC: World Bank; 2016.

16. World Health Organization. *National Systems to Support Drinking-Water, Sanitation and Hygiene: Global Status Report 2019. UN-Water Global Analysis and Assessment of Sanitation and Drinking-Water (GLAAS) 2019 Report*. Geneva: WHO; 2019.

17. Hutton G, Rodriguez U-P, Winara A, et al. *Economic Assessment of Sanitation Interventions in Southeast Asia*. Washington, DC: World Bank; 2014.

18. McGranahan G. Realizing the right to sanitation in deprived urban communities: Meeting the challenges of collective action, coproduction, affordability, and housing tenure. *World Development* 2014; *68*: 242–53.

19. Jamison D, Gelband H, Horton S, et al. DCP3: Disease Control Priorities. 2018. http://dcp-3.org (accessed 7 January 2021).

20. Hauck K, Martin S, Smith PC. Priorities for action on the social determinants of health: Empirical evidence on the strongest associations with life expectancy in 54 low-income countries, 1990–2012. *Social Science and Medicine* 2016; *167*: 88–98.

21. GBD Diarrhoeal Diseases Collaborators. Estimates of global, regional, and national morbidity, mortality, and aetiologies of diarrhoeal diseases: A systematic analysis for the Global Burden of Disease Study 2015. *Lancet Infectious Diseases* 2018; *17*: 909–48.

22. Keusch GT, Walker CF, Das JK, Horton S, Habte D. Diarrheal diseases. In: Black RE, Walker N, Laxminarayan R, Temmerman M, eds. *Reproductive, Maternal, Newborn, and Child Health*. 3rd edn. Washington, DC: International Bank for Reconstruction and Development/The World Bank; 2016: 163–86.
23. Waldman RJ, Mintz ED, Papowitz HE. The cure for cholera—improving access to safe water and sanitation. *New England Journal of Medicine* 2013; *368*: 592–4.
24. Montgomery M, Jones MW, Kabole I, Johnston R, Gordon B. No end to cholera without basic water, sanitation and hygiene. *Bulletin of the World Health Organization* 2018; *96*: 371–371A.
25. Dreibelbis R, Jenkins M, Chase RP, et al. Development of a multidimensional scale to assess attitudinal determinants of sanitation uptake and use. *Environmental Science & Technology* 2015; *49*: 13613–21.
26. Novotny J, Hasman J, Lepic M. Contextual factors and motivations affecting rural community sanitation in low- and middle-income countries: A systematic review. *International Journal of Hygiene and Environmental Health* 2018; *221*: 121–33.
27. Chambers R, Myers J. *Norms, Knowledge and Usage. Frontiers of CLTS: Innovations and Insights*. Brighton: Institute of Development Studies; 2016.
28. Hanchett S. Sanitation in Bangladesh: revolution, evolution, and new challenges. In: Bongartz P, Vernon N, Fox J, eds. *Sustainable Sanitation for All*. Rugby, UK: Practical Action Publishing; 2016: 31–52.
29. Coffey D, Gupta A, Hathi P, Spears D, Srivastav N, Vyas S. Understanding open defecation in rural India. Untouchability, pollution, and latrine pits. *Economic & Political Weekly* 2017; *52*: 59–66.
30. Coffey D, Spears D, Vyas S. Switching to sanitation: Understanding latrine adoption in a representative panel of rural Indian households. *Social Science and Medicine* 2017; 188: 41–50.
31. Gupta A, Coffey D, Spears D. Purity, pollution, and untouchability: Challenges affecting the adoption, use, and sustainability of sanitation programmes in rural India. In: Bongartz P, Vernon N, Fox J, eds. *Sustainable Sanitation for All*. Rugby, UK: Practical Action Publishing; 2016: 283–98.
32. Thomas A. Strengthening post-ODF programming: Reviewing lessons from sub-Saharan Africa. In: Bongartz P, Vernon N, Fox J, eds. *Sustainable Sanitation for All*. Rugby, UK: Practical Action Publishing; 2016: 83–97.
33. Kullmann C, Ahmed R. *Long Term Sustainability of Improved Sanitation in Rural Bangladesh*. Washington, DC: The Water and Sanitation Program; 2012.
34. Vernon N, Bongartz P. Going beyond open defecation free. In: Bongartz P, Vernon N, Fox J, eds. *Sustainable Sanitation for All*. Rugby, UK: Practical Action Publishing; 2016: 1–28.
35. Sinha A, Nagel CL, Schmidt WP, et al. Assessing patterns and determinants of latrine use in rural settings: A longitudinal study in Odisha, India. *International Journal of Hygiene and Environmental Health* 2017; *220*: 906–15.
36. Patil SR, Arnold BF, Salvatore AL, et al. The effect of India's total sanitation campaign on defecation behaviors and child health in rural Madhya Pradesh: A cluster randomized controlled trial. *PLoS Medicine* 2014; *11*: e1001709.

37. Czerniewska A, Muangi WC, Aunger R, Massa K, Curtis V. Theory-driven formative research to inform the design of a national sanitation campaign in Tanzania. *PloS One* 2019; *14*: e0221445.
38. Seleman A, Bhat MG. Multi-criteria assessment of sanitation technologies in rural Tanzania: Implications for program implementation, health and socio-economic improvements. *Technology in Society* 2016; *46*: 70–9.
39. Magalhaes Filho FJC, de Queiroz A, Machado BS, Paulo PL. Sustainable sanitation management tool for decision making in isolated areas in Brazil. *International Journal of Environmental Research and Public Health* 2019; *16*: 1–13.
40. Harvey PA. Environmental sanitation crisis: More than just a health issue. *Environmental Health Insights* 2008; *2*: 77–81.
41. Galvin M. Talking shit: Is community-led total sanitation a radical and revolutionary approach to sanitation? *WIREs Water* 2015; *2*: 9–20.
42. Nations U. *The Human Right to Water and Sanitation.* New York: United Nations; 2010.
43. Zaidi A. *From the Lane to the City: The Impact of the Orangi Pilot Project's Low Cost Sanitation Model.* London: Water Aid; 2001.
44. Hawkins P, Blackett I, Heymans C. *Poor-Inclusive Urban Sanitation: An Overview.* Washington, DC: The Water and Sanitation Program; 2013.
45. Saravanan VS. *'Blame it on the Community, Immunize the State and the International Agencies.' An Assessment of Water Supply and Sanitation Programs in India.* Bonn: ZEF; 2013.
46. Ostrom E. Crossing the great divide: Coproduction, synergy, and development. *World Development* 1996; *24*: 1073–87.
47. Northover H, Ryu SK, Brewer T. *Achieving Total Sanitation and Hygiene Coverage within a Generation—Lessons from East Asia.* Water Aid; 2016.
48. World Bank. *When Water Becomes a Hazard: A Diagnostic Report on the State of Water Supply, Sanitation, and Poverty in Pakistan and Its Impact on Child Stunting.* WASH Poverty Diagnostic Series, Washington, DC: World Bank; 2018.
49. Ronda RA. Pasig River Rehabilitation Commission gets international award. The Philippine Star. 19 October 2018.
50. Tiglao RD. Duterte must clean up the bigger 'cesspool' near his office—the Pasig River. The Manila Times. 2018 April 9.
51. World Bank. *Promising Progress: A Diagnostic of Water Supply, Sanitation, Hygiene, and Poverty in Bangladesh.* WASH Poverty Diagnostic. Washington, DC: World Bank, 2018.
52. Bryce J, Victora CG, Black RE. The unfinished agenda in child survival. *Lancet* 2013; *382*: 1049–59.
53. Copenhagen Consensus. Post-2015 consensus. Smart development goals. www.copenhagenconsensus.com/post-2015-consensus (accessed 7 January 2021). Copenhagen Consensus, 2015.
54. United Nations. Transforming our world: the 2030 Agenda for Sustainable Development. https://sustainabledevelopment.un.org/post2015/transforming-ourworld (accessed 7 January 2021).

55. United Nations. Sustainable Development Goal 6. Ensure availability and sustainable management of water and sanitation for all. https://sustainabledevelopment.un.org/sdg6 (accessed 7 January 2021).
56. Milan BF. Clean water and sanitation for all: Interactions with other sustainable development goals. *Sustainable Water Resources Management* 2017; *3*: 479–89.
57. Andersson K, Otoo M, Nolasco M. Innovative sanitation approaches could address multiple development challenges. *Water Science & Technology* 2018; *77*: 855–8.
58. Trimmer JT, Cusick RD, Guest JS. Amplifying progress toward multiple development goals through resource recovery from sanitation. *Environmental Science & Technology* 2017; *51*: 10765–76.
59. Black M, Fawcett B. *The Last Taboo: Opening the Door on the Global Sanitation Crisis.* London: Earthscan; 2008.
60. Koottatep T, Cookey PE, Polprasert C. (eds). *Regenerative sanitation: A new paradigm for sanitation 4.0.* London: IWA Publishing; 2019.
61. Langergraber G, Muellegger E. Ecological sanitation—a way to solve global sanitation problems? *Environment International* 2005; *31*: 433–44.

8
Our children's children

Hell is truth seen too late.

Thomas Adam (*Private Thoughts on Religion*, 1814)

Thomas Adam meant his dark warning to be taken literally, but it is an apt metaphor for the threat of disastrous climate change. An avoidable catastrophe might be allowed to happen if the danger is thought to be small, if the risk is low or uncertain, if it is remote in space or time, and if the cost of preventing it is high (Chapter 2). Those conditions help to explain why action on climate change has so far been slow.

But the magnitude of the climate threat is growing, in fact and in perception. From month to month, the risks and hazards linked to climate change—air pollution, drought, food shortages, floods, heatwaves, infectious diseases, storms, and wildfires—are becoming clearer, greater, and nearer. In the context of prevention, the challenge is to explain why it is worth paying sooner to avoid the costs of remedial action later—why we should put a high value on the future, today.

The preceding case studies (Chapters 3–7) have focused on aspects of health that are specific, temporary, or local. Climate change is a far bigger challenge to health and well-being because its effects will be wide-ranging, long-term, and global. This chapter asks how the principles of prevention (Chapter 2) can help to identify incentives for mitigating the causes and adapting to the consequences of climate change. Health is at the centre of this narrative (because it is the subject of this book), but human health contributes to, and profits from, healthy economies, environments, and societies, as set out in the 2030 Agenda for Sustainable Development.

The Great Health Dilemma. Christopher Dye, Oxford University Press. © Oxford University Press 2021.
DOI: 10.1093/oso/9780198853824.003.0008

Climate change

The essential facts about climate change are well known. In brief, the world is warming due to emissions of greenhouse gases (GHGs), predominantly carbon dioxide (CO_2), generated by combustion (fossil fuels, charcoal, wood), by anaerobic decomposition (wetlands, rice paddies), and from livestock (belching, manure). GHGs trap heat in the atmosphere, which in turn warms the land and oceans, thawing permafrost, acidifying and deoxygenating the seas, and melting polar ice and glaciers. Burning fossil fuels pushes up CO_2 concentrations in the atmosphere that will remain high for centuries, long after the fossil fuel era.

Besides CO_2, the other principal GHGs are methane (from natural gas, livestock manure, mining, rice cultivation, solid waste, and wastewater treatment), nitrous oxide (from fertilizers, fossil fuels, nitric acid production), tropospheric ozone (from sunlight-driven chemical reactions), black carbon (soot) and chloro- and hydrofluoro-carbons (used in air conditioners and refrigerators). In contrast to CO_2 and other long-lived GHGs (nitrous oxide has a half-life of around 120 years), methane, black carbon, tropospheric ozone and fluorinated gases are 'short-lived climate pollutants' (SLCPs), persisting in the atmosphere for periods ranging from a few days to a few years. SLCPs exist at much lower concentrations than CO_2 and can be removed more quickly, but they have greater 'global warming potential' (GWP) (e.g. the GWP of methane is 28–36 times greater than CO_2).

CO_2 emissions increased more or less continuously between 1960 and 2019 (Figure 8.1). The global atmospheric CO_2 concentration exceeded 400 parts per million in 2015—higher than ever previously experienced by humanity. CO_2 emissions are set to increase further despite scientific consensus that emissions must be sharply reduced if the global temperature is to be held to 2°C (and preferably 1.5°C) above pre-industrial levels, in line with the 2015 Paris Agreement (under the United Nations Framework Convention on Climate Change; Figure 8.1).[1,2] 'Committed' emissions from existing fossil fuel assets in the power, industrial, and transport sectors, together with inadequate national decarbonization plans, mean that the world is far from a trajectory that will prevent the global temperature from rising by more than 2°C.[3]

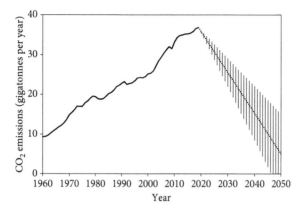

Figure 8.1 The huge challenge of cutting CO_2 emissions to stabilize global temperature. CO_2 production increased more or less continuously over the period 1960–2019 (line). To keep global temperature rise to less than 1.5°C above pre-industrial levels, emissions must turn sharply downwards from 2020 onwards, following a pathway somewhere within the shaded area (with variation depending on the climate model used).

Source: Data from Intergovernmental Panel on Climate Change. Global Warming of 1.5°C, an IPCC special report on the impacts of global warming of 1.5°C above pre-industrial levels and related global greenhouse gas emission pathways, in the context of strengthening the global response to the threat of climate change, sustainable development, and efforts to eradicate poverty. Geneva: Intergovernmental Panel on Climate Change, 2018.

Energy supplies

Fossil fuels still provide most of the world's energy. The contribution of coal to 'total final energy consumption' (TFEC) had stabilized by 2018 (27% of TFEC), but demand for oil (31%) and natural gas (23%) continued to increase. Pathways to decarbonization have been mapped out over the past two decades, using a combination of renewable energy technologies to replace fossil fuels—solar, wind, hydroelectric, geothermal and nuclear.[4–7] Although the cost of energy from renewable sources is falling quickly, the uptake is slow: by 2018, renewable energy (excluding traditional use of biomass) accounted for only 11% of TFEC, a small increase from around 10% in 2013. While some technologies are now familiar (solar and wind power, electric vehicles), other low-carbon innovations (heat pumps, household energy-saving devices) are still relatively expensive or unknown to the public at large.

Cheaper and more efficient renewable energy technologies (e.g. for carbon capture and storage) are still highly desirable, but the dominant challenge now is to implement the carbon-cutting solutions that already exist. The principal obstacles to producing energy cleanly are no longer technological but rather economic, political, institutional, and cultural.[7-11]

The COVID-19 pandemic has been an obstacle and an opportunity for the production of clean energy. Amid a global downturn in energy use during 2020, diminished investment has slowed the expansion of clean energy technologies.[12] On the other hand, renewables have proved to be the most resilient energy source as COVID-19 has spread worldwide. While the consumption of energy from coal, oil, gas, and nuclear sources has fallen in 2020, more electricity has been generated from wind turbines and solar plants, partly because electricity from these sources is delivered preferentially through power grids.[12]

The magnitude of the change in energy use during 2020 has underlined the huge challenge set by the 2015 Paris Agreement. Despite unprecedented lockdowns worldwide, energy-related carbon emissions are expected to fall by only 4%–7% during 2020. To keep the temperature imcrease under 1.5°C, emissions must continue to fall at least as quickly each year for the next 30 years (Figure 8.1).

From 2021 onwards, the rate of investment in clean energy will depend on public, political, and commercial incentives for mitigation and adaptation. From the perspective of government, holding a mirror to public opinion, a combination of prices, regulations, subsidies, services, and information will influence whether there is a collective will to 'build back better'.[13,14] COVID-19 is an opportunity-in-waiting: directing just a small fraction of pandemic recovery funds (US$12 trillion as of October 2020) to clean energy would contribute significantly to meeting the goals set in Paris in 2015.[15]

Costs and benefits for health

The diverse hazards of climate change affect health directly and indirectly.[16,17] The direct effects include illness, injury, and death from air pollution, droughts, floods, heatwaves, storms, and wildfires. The indirect effects operate via most of the pathways that link health to the Sustainable Development Goals (SDGs)—through poverty, undernutrition and overweight, inadequate sanitation, disrupted health services, homelessness and forced migration, social and economic inequality, among others.[18] The SDGs represent a health system in the broadest sense—a network of pathways defining mutual dependencies between health (SDG 3), climate change (SDG 13) and the other 15 Goals.[19]

The World Health Organization (WHO) calculated that there could be 250,000 additional deaths each year due to climate change between 2030 and 2050, from causes including heat stress, dengue, diarrhoeal diseases, malaria, and childhood undernutrition.[20] But this is no more than a starting point for analysis: considering all the direct and indirect effects together, the total impact on health is likely to be far greater.

Consequently, there are potentially large benefits for health from removing the risks. Mitigation, for example, can benefit health through agriculture (low-meat, plant-rich diets), transport (lower vehicle emissions, active travel), air quality (low-emission stoves), energy supply (power from renewable sources), and waste management (improved water treatment; Table 8.1).[16,21-23] These are pathways, not only for prevention (protecting health from climate change) but also to promote better health in the short and long run.

Among mitigation methods, the benefits of improving air quality are especially large. Ambient air pollution, including long- and short-lived GHGs and fine particulate matter, is the most important environmental cause of illness and death (2.94 million deaths in 2017, up from 1.75 million deaths in 1990). Household air pollution is also responsible for many deaths, though the number is falling each year (1.64 million in 2017, down from 2.71 million deaths in 1990).[24] Air pollution affects nearly every organ in the body, contributing to a wide variety of illnesses—acute lower respiratory infections, chronic obstructive pulmonary disease (COPD), ischaemic (coronary) heart disease, lung cancer, and stroke.

Cutting air pollution improves health quickly. In Ireland, a ban on indoor smoking reduced minor ailments within a few weeks: breathing difficulties, cough, phlegm, irritated eyes, painful throat, nasal itch, runny nose, sneeze, and wheeze. Just as quickly, there were measurable reductions in COPD, ischaemic heart disease, stroke, and all-cause mortality. Likewise, a variety of health and social benefits were reported within weeks of closing a steel mill in Utah: fewer people with respiratory illnesses, fewer premature births, and fewer school absentees. Within two months of the 2008 Beijing Olympics, lung function improved among healthy and asthmatic adults, there were fewer doctors' visits by asthma patients, and fewer deaths from cardiovascular diseases. In Nigeria, clean cooking stoves brought health

Table 8.1 Health gains from selected methods of climate change mitigation, with a classification of the potential for success. The full list also includes mitigation from industrial and waste products.

Mitigation method	Potential for CO_2 reduction	Certainty of major effect on short-lived climate pollutants	Potential health benefit	Main health benefits: direct, indirect or ancillary
Energy supply and electricity				
Switch from fossil fuels to renewable energy for large scale power production	High (coal, oil) or medium (gas)	Low	High (coal, oil) Low–medium (gas)	• Less crop damage and extreme weather • Improved air quality • Fewer occupational injuries
Transport				
Support for active and rapid mass transport	High	High	High	• Less crop damage and extreme weather • Improved air quality • Increased physical activity; reduced noise • Fewer traffic injuries
Agriculture				
Promotion of healthy diets low in processed and red meats and rich in plant-based foods	Medium–high	High	High	• Less crop damage and extreme weather • Reduced obesity and dietary diseases
Household air pollution and building design				
Low-emission stoves and/or reducing solid fuel use	Medium	Medium–high	High	• Less crop damage and extreme weather • Improved air quality • Lower risk of violence and injury during fuel collection

Source: World Health Organization (WHO). *COP24 Special Report: Health and Climate Change*. Geneva: WHO; 2019.

benefits within the term of a pregnancy: higher birthweights, fewer premature births, and reduced perinatal mortality.[25]

Actions are driven by perceptions as well as facts. Consequently, certain environmental effects on health attract greater attention and provoke a swifter response than others. One survey of US news networks found that stories about food shortages (some of which are linked to climate change) were included in only 3% of news bulletins, whereas earthquakes featured in 30% of bulletins, despite the far greater number of deaths linked to hunger than to seismic events.[26] Food shortages are more likely to stimulate action when the impersonal statistics of malnutrition are translated into personal stories about hunger and starvation.[10] The greater public concern about natural disasters may help to explain why the fatality rate has fallen markedly over the past century. There are no fewer disasters nowadays, but the number of deaths has fallen from millions in some years during the twentieth century to an average of 60,000 per year over the past decade.[27]

Professional judgements about the effects of climate change are as important as public perceptions. The economic gains from better health—obtained by meeting goals set by the 2015 Paris Agreement—would, according to one analysis, more than cover the global financial cost of mitigation: the value of the health gains, especially by improving air quality, would be approximately twice the cost of the policies, and a greater multiple in China and India.[16] But whether such arguments can tip the balance in favour of more aggressive climate mitigation, as WHO has suggested,[16] depends on how they are seen by the multi-trillion dollar energy industry.

Mitigation: Primary prevention

The singular advantage of mitigation is that climate change has one main cause—GHGs produced by burning fossil fuels for electricity, heating and transportation. Furthermore, most fossil fuels are extracted and sold by just a few big energy companies: between 1988 and 2015, 71% of GHG emissions came from fuels sold by 100 firms dominated by the 'Carbon Majors'—Chevron, ExxonMobil, Royal Dutch Shell, and BP, who were at that time continuing to develop new oil and gas fields.[28]

The single main cause, and the small number of perpetrators, point to a principal target for action—the price of carbon. Pricing mechanisms, most powerfully taxes on emissions, can effectively control supply and demand, provided governments are willing and able to use them (Chapter 6).[29] The goal of a carbon tax is to set a price for producers and consumers that reflects all the costs and benefits of GHGs to the economy, environment, and society, including health.[30] There is usually a gap—for example, between the full cost of vehicle fuel and the price paid by the consumer at the pump. That gap is, in effect, a subsidy to the motorist, although the subsidy might later be devalued by poor health linked to air pollution.[31] Raising the price of carbon lowers fuel consumption, cuts the emission of GHGs, and reduces illness due to air pollution.[32]

Whether taxes can be used effectively depends on the balance of arguments for and against. In their favour, taxes encourage energy consumers and producers to buy and sell less carbon-based fuel, by using less or by switching to cleaner energy. Governments should be enthusiastic about taxes because revenues can, in principle, be reinvested in managing climate change on behalf of taxpayers.

On the other hand, both producers and consumers might resist immediate price increases that are intended to pay for longer-term environmental and health benefits. For consumers especially, carbon taxes tend to be regressive, penalizing those for whom changes in fuel use are least affordable or convenient (this assumes that fuel is a necessity; cf. tobacco and sugar taxes; Chapter 6).

And consumers with tight budgets have an extra reason to reject higher fuel prices: they get little reward for their contribution to mitigation. Managing common, transnational resources, such as low atmospheric GHG concentrations, stable temperatures, glaciers, and polar ice sheets, needs coordinated action across countries.[33] The inhabitants of small island nations, for example, who cannot easily influence global climate change may decide that their money is better spent on local adaptation.

Despite political rhetoric about taking the long view ('our children's children' is the cliché), consumer preferences influence political decisions made on short electoral cycles where, among other things, relief is favoured over preparedness—cure over prevention. Prevention's perennial predicament is that voters are more inclined to reward leadership in the wake of a disaster rather than foresight in preparing for one (Chapter 2).[31] Former president of the European Commission, Jean-Claude Juncker, spoke on behalf of many a well-meaning politician: 'We all know what to do, but we don't know how to get re-elected once we have done it.'

In aggregate, the perceived benefits of carbon taxes for environment and health do not yet outweigh the costs—the price of carbon is too low. As of 2018, only 14% of global GHG emissions were covered by carbon-pricing mechanisms, and the global emissions-weighted price per tonne of CO_2 dropped from a high of US\$50 in 2000 to US\$15 in 2018.[34] Over the same period, state subsidies to energy companies for fossil fuel production rose to a high of US\$430 billion. For global emissions that were covered by carbon-pricing mechanisms in 2018, less than 5% of were priced at a level that would satisfy the ambitions of the 2015 Paris Agreement; that is, US\$40–80/tonne CO_2 by 2020 and US\$50–100/tonne CO_2 by 2030.[35]

Further progress on carbon pricing can be made by studying specific successes and failures. In 2017, Chile began to apply green taxes on companies emitting local (fine particulate matter, nitrous oxide, sulphur dioxide) and global pollutants (CO_2). Air pollution was seen as the country's foremost environmental problem.[36] Based on the 'polluter pays' principle, and a sense of common responsibility, taxes were presented as corrective rather than punitive. Tax levies were adjusted to charge the social cost of the damage generated, thereby giving incentives to switch to cleaner technologies. The deeper question—not answered by the bare facts—is why the government of Chile was willing and able to introduce green taxes when other governments have not been able to do so.

French government proposals to raise fuel (especially diesel) prices in 2018 were dropped after weeks of public protest in 2018. A lesson from France is that context and timing are critical: street protests steered by the 'gilets jaunes' (yellow vests) movement were only partly about carbon taxes: they were also motivated by government policies on wealth taxes and the minimum wage, by rising costs and falling living standards (cf. France's more successful approach to tobacco taxation; Chapter 6).

Clearly, carbon taxes alone will not be sufficient to mitigate climate change, so other measures are needed. The options for government include cap and trade systems for carbon emissions; ending subsidies for coal, oil, and gas production, to be replaced with subsidies for wind, solar, and hydropower; creating higher standards for energy efficiency; and investing in public transport.

There are key roles, too, for institutions and organizations outside government. Judicial procedures are notoriously slow but the role of litigation is growing in climate change mitigation (and adaptation). Medical and legal systems use different criteria to judge the strength of evidence linking cause and effect. So the standard criteria for establishing a causal link—for example, between environment and disease—need to be interpreted alongside, for instance, the 'balance of probability' and 'beyond reasonable doubt' as used in law.[37]

By 2020, the Grantham Research Institute had logged more than 1,900 pieces of climate legislation worldwide, about two-thirds enacted in the preceding decade. At least 37 countries and eight regional and international jurisdictions had reported one or more lawsuits related to climate change; 80% were brought against governments, mainly by corporations or individuals.[38] Climate change was at the centre of the legal argument in 41%. The majority (and 58% of those outside the US) had outcomes favouring mitigation or adaptation. A growing number of cases were underpinned by arguments on human rights, as specified by the 2015 Paris Agreement.

Strengthening arguments for accountability, 'attribution science' is extending methods of inferring causality: providing evidence that attributes specific effects—for example, on health or environment—to their determinants.[39] It is increasingly possible to attribute droughts, floods, hurricanes, and wildfires to GHG emissions, and then to the agencies responsible.[40–42] Europe's 2003 heatwave caused around 27,000 excess deaths. The first 'extreme event attribution' study found it to be 'very likely' (>90%) that human influence at least doubled the risk of that heatwave.[43]

It is not possible to prove that human-induced environmental change damaged the health of a particular individual, but a court of law might accept that it has, considering the weight of evidence.[37] Nine-year old Ella Kissi-Debrah is a case in point. Living close to the South Circular Road in Lewisham, London, she was exposed to consistently high levels of air pollution. She suffered a fatal asthma attack in February 2013 after three years of seizures and many hospital visits for breathing problems. In 2019, a London court made a provisional ruling to carry out a full inquest into her death under the Human Rights Act. In December 2020, a coroner determined, in a landmark ruling, that air pollution was indeed a cause of her death. He decided that air pollution both induced and exacerbated Ella's form of severe asthma. This ruling will undoubtedly increase pressure on the UK government to reduce illegal levels of air pollution across the country (cf. glyphosate weed killer as a cause of cancer; Chapter 2).[44]

Adaptation: Secondary prevention

Given the huge challenge of making large and rapid reductions in GHG emissions (Figure 8.1), mitigation will necessarily be supported by adaptation.[9]

Adaptation (downstream, secondary prevention) is inferior to mitigation (upstream, primary prevention) in the sense that its effects are remedial and relatively small in scale. On the other hand, the incentives are clear: adaptation responds to specific and predictable local threats, with interventions that are likely to provide rapid returns on investment. An extra advantage is that it is not necessary to ascertain that climate change is the underlying cause of droughts, fires, and floods before deciding to take action. Furthermore, many forms of adaptation, particularly in cities, are under the control of local authorities that provide, independently of national governments, a large proportion of energy, transport, water, sanitation, and health services.[16]

Climate change adaptation is a growth industry, but still in its formative stages. An average of US$579 billion per year was spent on climate change in 2017 and 2018, but only US$30 billion (5.2%) was allocated to adaptation, mostly from public rather than private funds.[47]

Financial support for adaptations that benefit health is also low: about 5% of all funding for adaptation in 2017.[21] A survey of global multilateral funds that support adaptation found that only US$9 million (0.5%) of more than US$1.5 billion was allocated to projects that address health, despite appeals for support from the health ministers of vulnerable countries.[16]

As with mitigation, successful adaptation depends on resolving competing interests. In 2018, monsoon flooding killed at least 400 people in Kerala state, India, and left a million people homeless.[48] In Kerala, as elsewhere, adaptation depends on understanding why illegal stone quarrying, deforestation, and construction, all of which exacerbated the flooding, were permitted to breech environmental laws.[49]

Where mitigation fails, adaptation is a necessity. The number of adaptation projects has been increasing in European countries since 2006 onwards (Figure 8.2).[45] More projects have been established at local than at national level and, as expected, these projects were tailored to local needs—the prevention of extreme urban temperatures, flooding, and water scarcity, among others.

Tipping points: Triggers for action

Gradual change breeds hesitation in the face of a slowly evolving emergency.[50,51] As psychologist Daniel Gilbert put it: 'Many environmentalists say climate change is happening too fast. No, it's happening too

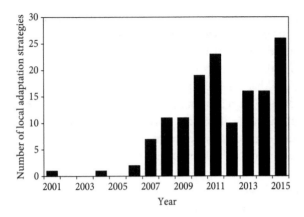

Figure 8.2 The growing number of local (sub-national) strategies for climate change adaptation in European countries, 2001–15.

Adapted from Aguiar, F.C., Bentza, J., Silva, J.M.N., *et al.* (2018). Adaptation to climate change at local level in Europe: An overview. Environmental Science and Policy, 86: 38–63; European Climate Adaptation Platform Climate-ADAPT. Climate Adapt. Copyright (c) 2018 American Chemical Society.

slowly.[52] There are plenty of supporting data: a 2018 study by the European Environment Agency examined 88 slow-moving environmental problems; in 84 of these cases, policy inaction allowed problems to worsen despite years of warnings.[51]

Shock is a remedy for prevarication. Possible 'tipping points' in the geo-physical climate system mean that there is potential for abrupt, non-linear, irreversible changes, such as the collapse of the West Antarctic ice sheet or a rapid switch from rainforests to savannas.[53] Worse still, exceeding a threshold in one system (ice sheets) could heighten the risk of crossing boundaries in others (deserts, ocean currents, forests), with cascading effects between physical and ecological systems. A consistent finding of climate analysis is that the hazards are great and the risks are high. The impacts, if not already here, are coming soon, and perhaps more quickly than expected.

In their discussion of abrupt changes to the climate system, Timothy Lenton and colleagues adapted utility theory (Chapter 2) to define an emergency (E) as: the risk that an event will happen, multiplied by the size of the hazard (damage caused, H), and by the reaction time to a future event (τ) divided by the time left to prevent it (T). Thus, $E = pH\tau/T$.[53]

In the context of climate change, this formula needs further elaboration (as does the theory outlined in Chapter 2). The modification would capture the potential for tipping points both in the development of an emergency (a sudden change in p, H or T) and in the response to it (events that precipitate urgent action, shortening τ).

Although some commentators see a long and arduous road ahead,[3,54] others have identified 'sensitive intervention points' where 'a small kick ... may have an outsized effect', causing rapid change in the social, financial, and political systems that govern action on climate change.[55,56]

While observing all necessary cautions (climate pledges have a chequered history), it is clear that business is becoming increasingly sensitive to the threat posed by climate change and other man-made environmental disasters, as reflected in recent annual reports of the World Economic Forum (Figure 8.3). In the energy industry, a growing fear of 'stranded assets' (fossil fuels priced or regulated out of use) is forcing a switch from strategies that wantonly impede decarbonization to strategies that capitalize on the inevitable and imminent change. Decarbonization is becoming the shrewd business choice—achieved by selling dirty assets, buying cleaner energy, investing in low-carbon products, and decarbonizing supply chains.[57]

Principles for Responsible Investment, an investors group with trillions of dollars under management, predicts 'abrupt and disruptive' climate policies by 2025.[59] Their 'inevitable policy response' sees oil demand peak as soon as 2026–28. Wind and solar power will generate half the world's electricity by 2030. Coal, the most carbon-polluting fossil fuel, will be 'virtually non-existent' by 2040. Petrol and diesel vehicles will be phased out more quickly than forecasted by others, and forestation will be greatly accelerated.

One of Europe's biggest oil and gas firms, Repsol, agrees. Repsol was the first major oil company to set a target of net zero carbon emissions by 2050.[60] Royal Dutch Shell proposes to cut CO_2 emissions by its consumers by 20% before 2035, and to set specific targets for three- to five-year periods from 2020 onwards. Shell also intends to link emissions targets to executive pay.[61] BP's 'Rapid' change scenario imagines a 70% reduction in carbon emissions from energy use between 2018 and 2050, keeping the rise in global temperature to less than 2°C, driven by a substantial increase in carbon prices.[62]

Following suit, the world's largest asset manager, BlackRock, announced in 2020 that it will divest more than half a billion US dollars in coal shares from all of its actively managed portfolios.[63] In their view, climate change

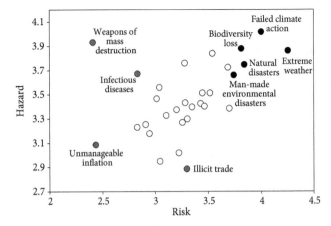

Figure 8.3 The Global Risks Perception Survey (2020) compiled for the World Economic Forum (WEF). Five of the top threats (large hazard, high risk; black circles) to business, government, and civil society were associated with environmental and climate change. Among the other threats (grey circles) were infectious diseases (evaluated before COVID-19) and weapons of mass destruction (large hazard, low risk), illicit trade (tax evasion, human trafficking, organized crime; small hazard, moderate risk) and unmanageable inflation (small hazard, low risk). Risk is termed 'likelihood' and hazard is labelled 'impact' by WEF, adjusted here for consistency in this book. Risk is the probability of occurrence over the next 10 years; hazard is the severity of the impact at global level, each ranked on a scale 1–5.

Adapted with permission from World Economic Forum. The Global Risks Report 2020. Geneva: World Economic Forum, 2020.

must now be routinely factored into the risk of investment. Pension funds, too, are taking a stand against 'short-termism'. Japan's Government Pension Investment Fund believes that a focus on short-sighted returns leaves their portfolios open to 'potentially catastrophic systemic risks'. Their stated intent is, from now on, is to price in the environment and the long-term well-being of workers and communities.[64]

Insurance companies also face huge losses as extreme events become more frequent and more intense. In terms of insurance pay-outs, 2018 was the fourth-costliest year since 1980.[65] Although insurance instruments such as catastrophe bonds have a choppy history (Chapter 4), there are strong incentives for insurance companies to learn how to indemnify disasters; if they cannot do business in the face of catastrophes, billions of people will be left vulnerable to devastation.

Adding to the shift in mood among businesses, there is movement among signatories to the 2015 Paris Agreement. In 2019, the UK became the first large economy to pass a zero emissions law, requiring net zero GHG emissions by 2050.[66] The UK agriculture sector, which is responsible for around 9% of national GHG emissions, has also set a more ambitious goal: to achieve the UK target by 2040 by using robots to replace tractors, drones for precision pesticide application, tree planting, cutting soya feed for livestock, and lowering methane production by cattle through breeding and husbandry. Naturally, environmentalists want more and sooner, including low-meat and low-dairy diets. Nevertheless, the challenge of reducing GHG emissions has been accepted, not rejected, by agriculture, energy, and other sectors of the economy. At the UN General Assembly on 22 September 2020, President Xi Jinping announced that 'China will scale up its Intended Nationally Determined Contributions by adopting more vigorous policies and measures. We aim to have [carbon dioxide] emissions peak before 2030 and achieve carbon neutrality before 2060.'[67] Such a large, unilateral commitment from the world's biggest emitter of CO_2, if sincere, puts economic incentives and political pressures in front of other national governments.

There is little systematic information about how to generate transformative change,[68,69] but there are examples on which to build the knowledge base. Benjamin Sovacool has described a series of rapid transitions in the adoption of clean energy sources and technologies, which benefit health more and less directly.[70] During the 1990s, Sweden made a comprehensive shift to energy-efficient lighting in commercial buildings within a decade. To drive the change, the government directly purchased 30,000 lighting units in a pilot phase and supported their installation. They introduced technical standards and quality assurance, plus subsidies and methods for bulk purchase and procurement. Market penetration jumped from 10% in 1996 to almost 70% by 2000.

Between 1983 and 1998, China's National Improved Stove Program promoted the invention and distribution of energy-efficient cooking stoves, increasing coverage from 1% of the Chinese market to more than 80%, reaching half a billion people after 15 years.

From 2007 onwards, households in Indonesia received government help to convert cooking stoves from kerosene to liquefied petroleum gas (LPG) so as to improve air quality. A free starter package included a filled LPG cylinder and a burner stove. Kerosene subsidies were cut (pushing up the price) and new LPG terminals served as national distribution hubs. In just three years between 2007 and 2009, the number of LPG stoves nation-wide increased from 3 million to 43 million, reaching almost two-thirds of Indonesian households.

Brazil made two separate but rapid transitions from petrol to ethanol fuels for private cars. Beginning in 1975, the Proálcool programme scaled up production so that 90% of all new vehicles could run on ethanol by 1981. Then, in 2003, lower fuel taxes encouraged motorists to buy flex-fuel ve-hicles (FFVs), which could run on any blend of fuel, from zero to pure ethanol. FFV drivers could switch between various blends of gasoline and ethanol depending on price and convenience. FFV sales grew from 17% of new cars in 2004 to 90% in 2009.

Rapid changes in the primary source of energy are possible too. The decommissioning of coal-fired power plants in Ontario, Canada, beginning in 2003, was strongly motivated by public health. Eliminating coal would, it was estimated, cut pollution-related illnesses from 330,000 to fewer than 2,500 per year and nearly eliminate associated deaths, with an added eco-nomic dividend. To make the transition, the government of Ontario in-vested in hydroelectric, solar, wind, and nuclear power, in addition to improving the efficiency of energy distribution.

Although none of these selected success stories had a single cause, polit-ical leadership played a key role in most (as it has in sanitation; Chapter 7). From carbon taxes to cleaner cars, that leadership will be vital in seizing the opportunities for a rapid energy transition—the more so where there is continued resistance from fossil fuel lobbies, where public support is still tentative, and where financiers need greater confidence to invest in a low-carbon future.[71,72]

Summary

Climate change is prevention's biggest challenge—its effects on health and well-being will be wide-ranging, long-term, and global. The pressures and opportunities for action are growing as the risks and hazards become clearer, greater and nearer. Mitigation—cutting GHG emissions (primary prevention)—benefits health, economy, environment, and society through agriculture, transport, air quality, energy supply, and waste management. Adaptation (secondary prevention) is the essential back-up when miti-gation fails; there are strong incentives for local adaptation to counter predictable local threats such as extreme urban temperatures, flooding, and water scarcity. Carbon taxes are a powerful but underexploited mechanism for reducing GHG emissions, so need to be reinforced by other incentives, including subsidies for wind, solar, hydrogen, and hydropower. Now more than ever, the pressure for transformative action on climate change, embracing the health benefits, has the potential to stimulate sudden and rapid movement towards clean energy sources and technologies.

References

1. Intergovernmental Panel on Climate Change (IPCC). *Global Warming of 1.5°C: An IPCC Special Report on the Impacts of Global Warming of 1.5°C above Pre-Industrial Levels and Related Global Greenhouse Gas Emission Pathways, in the Context of Strengthening the Global Response to the Threat of Climate Change, Sustainable Development, and Efforts to Eradicate Poverty.* Geneva: IPCC; 2018.
2. Watts N, Gong P, Campbell-Lendrum D, Costello A, Robinson E. Health and climate change—Authors' reply. *Lancet* 2019; *393*: 2197–8.
3. Roberts C, Geels FW. Conditions for politically accelerated transitions: Historical institutionalism, the multi-level perspective, and two historical case studies in transport and agriculture. *Technological Forecasting & Social Change* 2019; *140*: 221–40.
4. Pacala S, Socolow R. Stabilization wedges: Solving the climate problem for the next 50 years with current technologies. *Science* 2004; *305*: 968–72.
5. Jacobson MZ, Delucchi MA, Cameron MA, et al. Impacts of green new deal energy plans on grid stability, costs, jobs, health, and climate in 143 countries. *One Health* 2019; *1*: 449–63.
6. Griffith S. The Green New Deal: The enormous opportunity in shooting for the moon. 2019. https://medium.com/otherlab-news/decarbonization-and-gnd-b8ddd569de16 (accessed 7 January 2021).
7. Griffith S. *Rewiring America: A Field Manual for the Climate Fight.* San Francisco, 2020.
8. Diesendorf M, Elliston B. The feasibility of 100% renewable electricity systems: A response to critics. *Renewable and Sustainable Energy Reviews* 2018; *93*: 318–30.
9. Global Commission on Adaptation. *Adapt Now: A Global Call for Leadership on Climate Resilience.* Rotterdam and Washington, DC: Global Center on Adaptation, World Resources Institute; 2019.
10. Marshall G. *Don't even Think about It: Why our Brains Are Wired to Ignore Climate Change.* New York: Bloomsbury; 2014.
11. Sovacool BK. The importance of comprehensiveness in renewable electricity and energy-efficiency policy. *Energy Policy* 2009; *37*: 1529–41.
12. IEA. Global Energy Review 2020. 2020. https://www.iea.org/ (accessed 7 January 2021).

13. Hepburn C, O'Callaghan B, Stern N, Stiglitz J, Zenghelis D. *Will COVID-19 Fiscal Recovery Packages Accelerate or Retard Progress on Climate Change?* Working paper no. 20-02. Oxford: Smith School of Enterprise and the Environment (SSEE); 2020.

14. IEA. World Energy Outlook 2020. 2020. https://www.iea.org/ (accessed 7 January 2021).

15. Andrijevic M, Schleussner CF, Gidden MJ, McCollum DL, Rogelj J. COVID-19 recovery funds dwarf clean energy investment needs. *Science* 2020; *370*: 298–300.

16. World Health Organization. *COP24 Special Report: Health and Climate Change.* Geneva: WHO; 2019.

17. World Health Organization. *COP24 Special Report: Health and Climate Change.* Geneva: WHO; 2018.

18. World Health Organization. *World Health Statistics 2020: Monitoring For The SDGs, Sustainable Development Goals.* Geneva: WHO; 2020.

19. Dye C. Expanded health systems for sustainable development. *Science* 2018; *359*: 1337–9.

20. World Health Organization. Fact sheets: climate change and health. 2018. https://www.who.int/news-room/fact-sheets/detail/climate-change-and-health (accessed 7 January 2021).

21. Watts N, Amann M, Arnell N, et al. The 2019 report of The Lancet Countdown on health and climate change: Ensuring that the health of a child born today is not defined by a changing climate. *Lancet* 2019; *394*: 1836–78.

22. European Academies Science Advisory Council. *The Imperative of Climate Action to Protect Human Health in Europe.* Halle: German National Academy of Sciences Leopoldina; 2019.

23. Haines A, Amann M, Borgford-Parnell N, Leonard S, Kuylenstierna J, Shindell D. Short-lived climate pollutant mitigation and the Sustainable Development Goals. *Nature Climate Change* 2017; *7*: 863–9.

24. Institute for Health Metrics and Evaluation (IHME). GBD results tool. 2020. http://ghdx.healthdata.org/gbd-results-tool (accessed 7 January 2021).

25. Schraufnagel DE, Balmes JR, De Matteis S, et al. Health benefits of air pollution reduction. *Annals of the American Thoracic Society* 2019; *16*: 1478–87.

26. Eisensee T, Strömberg D. News droughts, news floods, and US disaster relief. *The Quarterly Journal of Economics* 2007; *122*: 693–728.

27. Ritchie H et al. Statistics and research: Coronavirus pandemic (COVID–19). 2020. https://ourworldindata.org/coronavirus (accessed 7 January 2021).

28. Climate Accountability Institute. Carbon majors. 2019. https://climateaccountability.org/carbonmajors.html (accessed 7 January 2021).

29. Best R, Burke PJ, Jotzo F. Carbon pricing efficacy: Cross-country evidence. *Environmental and Resource Economics* 2020; *77*: 69–94.

30. Amadeo K. Carbon tax, its purpose, and how it works. 2020. https://www.thebalance.com/carbon-tax-definition-how-it-works-4158043 (accessed 7 January 2021).

31. Pigato MA, (ed.). *Fiscal Policies for Development and Climate Action.* Washington, DC: World Bank; 2019.

32. Parry I, Veung C, Heine D. *How much Carbon Pricing is in Countries' Own Interests? The Critical Role of Co-Benefits.* Munich: Centre for Economic Studies & Ifo Institute; 2014.
33. Boyd R, Richerson PJ, Meinzen-Dick R, et al. Tragedy revisited. *Science* 2018; *362*: 1236–41.
34. Ripple WJ. World scientists' warning of a climate emergency. *BioScience* 2019.
35. World Bank. *State and Trends of Carbon Pricing 2019.* Washington, DC: World Bank; 2019.
36. Pizarro R, Pinto F, Ainzúa S. *Chile's Green' Tax Strategy.* Santiago: Ministry of the Environment; 2017.
37. The Royal Society. *The Use of Statistics in Legal Proceedings: A Primer for Courts.* London: The Royal Society; 2020.
38. Setzer J, Byrnes R. *Global Trends in Climate Change Litigation: 2020 Snapshot.* London: Grantham Research Institute on Climate Change and the Environment and Centre for Climate Change Economics and Policy, London School of Economics and Political Science; 2020.
39. Allen M. Liability for climate change. *Nature* 2003; *421*: 891–2.
40. Colman Z. The new science fossil fuel companies fear. *Politico.* 22 October 2019.
41. Licker R, Ekwurzel B, Doney SC, et al. Attributing ocean acidification to major carbon producers. *Environmental Research Letters* 2019; *14*: 124060.
42. Vautard R, van Aalst M, Boucher O, et al. Human contribution to the record-breaking June and July 2019 heatwaves in Western Europe. *Environmental Research Letters* 2020; *15*: 094077.
43. Stott PA, Stone DA, Allen MR. Human contribution to the European heatwave of 2003. *Nature* 2004; *432*: 610–4.
44. The Guardian. Inquest to determine if London air pollution caused child's death. *The Guardian.* 17 December 2019.
45. Aguiar FC, Bentza J, Silva JMN, et al. Adaptation to climate change at local level in Europe: An overview. *Environmental Science and Policy* 2018; *86*: 38–63.
46. European Climate Adaptation Platform Climate-ADAPT. 2020. https://climate-adapt.eea.europa.eu (accessed 7 January 2021).
47. Climate Policy Initiative. *Global Landscape of Climate Finance 2019.* London: Climate Policy Initiative; 2019.
48. Guterres A. Secretary-General's remarks on climate change. 2018. https://www.un.org/sg/en/content/sg/statement/2018-09-10/secretary-generals-remarks-climate-change-delivered (accessed 7 January 2021).
49. India Today. Kerala floods is man-made calamity: Madhav Gadgil. India Today. 18 August 2018.
50. Barrett S, Dannenberg A. Sensitivity of collective action to uncertainty about climate tipping points. *Nature Climate Change* 2014; *4*: 36–9.
51. Olson RL, Rejeski D. Slow threats and environmental policy. *Environmental Law Reporter* 2018; *48*: 10116–24.
52. Gilbert D. *Global Warming and Psychology.* Cambridge, Mass.: Harvard University; 2010.
53. Lenton TM, Rockstrom J, Gaffney O, et al. Climate tipping points—too risky to bet against. *Nature* 2019; *575*: 592–5.

54. Smil V. *Energy Transitions: History, Requirements, Prospects.* Westport, CT:Preager; 2010.
55. Farmer JD, Hepburn C, Ives MC, et al. Sensitive intervention points in the post-carbon transition. *Science* 2019; *364*: 132–4.
56. Climate change: 'the Paris goals are within reach'. Financial Times 12 December 2020. https://www.ft.com/content/d6e23e40-2d6b-4e8c-b92b-6bf1b215798d
57. Scriven G. The great disrupter. The Economist. 2020.
58. World Economic Forum. *The Global Risks Report 2020.* Geneva: World Economic Forum; 2020.
59. Principles for Responsible Investment. *The Inevitable Policy Response.* London: Principles for Responsible Investment; 2019.
60. Vaughan A. Peak oil demand could arrive much sooner than expected, says oil firm. *New Scientist*, 4 January 2020.
61. Raval A, Hook L, Mooney A. Shell yields to investors by setting target on carbon footprint. Financial Times, 3 December 2018.
62. BP. *bp Energy Outlook 2020.* London: BP; 2020.
63. BlackRock. Thematic investing with BlackRock and iShares. 2020. https://www.blackrock.com/uk/intermediaries/themes/thematic-investing/explained (accessed 7 January 2021).
64. Lewis L, Patrick Temple-West P. Pension fund giants team up in attack on 'short-termism'. Financial Times. 4 March 2020.
65. Munich Re. The natural disasters of 2018 in figures. 2019. https://www.munichre.com/topics-online/en/climate-change-and-natural-disasters/natural-disasters/the-natural-disasters-of-2018-in-figures.html (accessed 7 January 2021).
66. The Sixth Carbon Budget. The UK's path to Net Zero. Committee on Climate Change. 2020.
67. Tooze A. How Xi just saved the world. *Foreign Policy*, 26 September 2020.
68. Tabara JD, Frantzeskaki N, Hoelscher K, et al. Positive tipping points in a rapidly warming world. *Current Opinion in Environmental Sustainability* 2018; *31*: 120–9.
69. Fisher S. Can we identify the tipping points for transformative climate action?: *Climate-KIC.* 20 June 2019.
70. Sovacool BK. How long will it take? Conceptualizing the temporal dynamics of energy transitions. *Energy Research & Social Science* 2016; *13*: 202–15.
71. Friel S. Climate change and the people's health: The need to exit the consumptagenic system. *Lancet.* 20 February 2020.
72. Climate Finance Leadership Initiative. *Financing the Low-Carbon Future: A Private-Sector View on Mobilizing Climate Finance.* New York: Climate Finance Leadership Initiative; 2019.

9
Future positive

The doctor of the future will give no medicine, but will interest his patient in the care of the human frame, in diet and in the cause and prevention of disease.

Thomas Edison (1903)

Twenty-two centuries after Pien Ch'iao (Chapter 1), Thomas Edison restated history's enduring ambition. But he must have realized, like many who came before and after, that we pay a price to care for the human frame—counted in money, time, effort, information, trust, and willpower. Consequently, the decision facing doctors and their patients is conditional: prevention is better than cure, but not at any price.

Another century on from Edison, this book's purpose has been to explore ways of reaching that still-imagined future. The argument rests on a simple proposition: understanding why people prefer to take a chance on sickness and cure is the key to persuading them when and why they should choose prevention instead. In public health, as in other fields, people are more likely to act on reasoned arguments rather than unjustified commandments.

Seeking motives instead of issuing directives, the history (Chapter 1), principles (Chapter 2), and case studies (Chapters 3–8) examine, not merely what should be done, but why anyone would choose to do it. The case studies have explored some of the obstacles to prevention, and how to overcome them, in the context of healthcare services (competing for resources), epidemics, and emergencies (managing risks), endemic infectious disease (perceived hazards), chronic, non-communicable diseases (constraints on choice), sanitation (social preferences), and climate change (valuing the future; Table 9.1). The purpose of comparing prevention in different settings is to identify the commonalities, among the details of specific applications.

The Great Health Dilemma. Christopher Dye, Oxford University Press. © Oxford University Press 2021.
DOI: 10.1093/oso/9780198853824.003.0009

Table 9.1 The problems of prevention: topics and themes, with selected obstacles and solutions, drawn from six case studies in Chapters 3-8

Topic	Main theme	Obstacles	Solutions
Health care services	Cost: competing for resources	• Health services are primarily for medical treatment, prevention is ancillary and low priority; no equivalent comprehensive service for prevention • Prevention outside health services is controlled by other sectors of government	• Protect the budget for prevention in health services, having assessed the full benefits • Define the health and other joint benefits of prevention across government sectors as a basis for health in all policies (HiAP)
Epidemics and emergencies	Risk: insurance for unlikely disasters	• Low and unpredictable risk of diverse, high-impact pathogens, some of which are unknown (Disease X) • Limited options for managing animal and environmental reservoirs • Prevention is low priority in emergencies	• Insurance mechanisms to pool risks and share costs through finance, technology platforms, and exchange of data and materials • Secondary prevention by surveillance, early detection, and rapid response to outbreaks • Invest in preparedness during 'peace time', with broad functions to cover all types of emergency
Endemic infectious diseases	Hazard: re-evaluating familiar threats	• Low perceived threat of predictable endemic disease • Low risk per capita even with large population burden of disease • No effective vaccines for tuberculosis (TB) and HIV/AIDS	• Highlight epidemic features of endemic disease, including new types of disease (e.g. drug resistance) and outbreaks in new locations • 'Treatment as prevention' cures illness and reduces mortality as well as interrupting transmission; reduce joint risk of TB and HIV/AIDS through antiretroviral therapy • Promising results of recent vaccine trials should boost research funding

Chronic (non-communicable) diseases	Choice: opting for healthier lifestyles	• Low perceived risk to individuals (among all other risks); slow onset of chronic diseases; limited choice and information to individuals at risk	• Government policies (taxes, regulations, subsidies, services, information) to facilitate public choice; large, rapid benefits of reducing major risks e.g. tobacco, sugar
Sanitation	Culture: aligning social preferences	• Sanitary behaviour depends on personal preferences and social norms • High costs of sanitation (e.g. infrastructure), not primarily for health; diverse sources of infection limit efficacy of single interventions	• Collective decisions to align the goals of providers (waste removal, health, energy) and consumers (sanitary practices) • Define interventions rather than diseases e.g. sanitation combined with animal husbandry, housing, food safety, vaccination, waste removal, to set full benefits against costs
Climate change	Time: valuing the future	• Uncertain risk, timing, and magnitude of adverse effects • Slow reaction to a slowly evolving threat • Impact not primarily on health	• Adapt (secondary prevention) to specific local threats, delivering rapid returns on investment • Exploit potential tipping points in social, economic, and political systems • Promote mitigation by adding health co-benefits to climate change accounting e.g. from less air pollution; invoke legal as well as medical arguments to safeguard health

Common principles, diverse practices

Prevention is a choice made in anticipation of the future. The ideas about how to make that choice focus here on health, but the principles have been developed and applied by specialists of all kinds, from actuaries to zoologists. The great health dilemma is a more general dilemma about making choices now, for the present and the future.

To make progress here, the principles are gathered together in a testable—and refutable—idea. The proposition is that the choices people make about health are rational: prevention is more likely to be favoured over cure when an imminent, high-risk, high-impact hazard can be averted at relatively low cost.

'Rational' just means that the choices, among the options available, are informed by judgement and reason: people make decisions on the basis of what is judged to be good and bad, personally, professionally, and for society. The reason for a decision may not be immediately obvious (apparently 'irrational') but will yield to investigation. Behavioural studies usually show that the decisions people make about health depend, not only on quantified costs, risks, and hazards, but also on the incentives, motives, powers, and values of everyone who has a stake in the outcome—individuals, governments, non-governmental organizations, businesses, and others. The stakeholders interact with one another, and the net effect on public health depends on their collective action (Chapter 2).

There is nothing conceptually new in this approach, which has its quantitative origins in eighteenth-century probability theory, and especially with Daniel Bernouilli's 1738 'expected utility hypothesis'. As with Bernouilli's hypothesis, the theory used here not intended to be a statement of truth but rather an efficient method of investigation—a framework for drawing together and testing the arguments for prevention in diverse settings. The latest discoveries, for example, in behavioural economics and finance, have emerged by testing and refining earlier ideas about how people make choices when faced with different options. In health as in other disciplines, some of the choices that have been described as illogical 'false economies' make sense in light of new discoveries about human behaviour (Chapter 2).

Qualitative application of these principles, together with the case studies, offers 12 lessons for prevention. They cover the main elements of choice identified throughout this book—hazard perception, risk management, time preference, cost saving, and the practical constraints on choice—but with some essential extras. The additions include methods for accounting and for introducing accountability; for defining the right questions about prevention; for promoting good health as well as preventing illness; for improving efficiency and for enabling cooperation. Some methods are oriented specifically to prevention (such as valuing the future); others apply to medical treatment too (including perceptions of hazard). Some have been stated before.[1] Collectively, they are based on a mix of promising ideas, instructive failures, and proven successes. And collectively, they set a large agenda for future research.

Twelve lessons for prevention

Positive economics

Mindful of the long history of health choices framed by contingency and circumstance (Chapter 1), investigations here give precedence to 'positive' over 'normative' economics: favouring description of 'what is' (leading to testable ideas about cause and effect) before prescribing 'what should be' (often based on unsupported value judgments).

To revisit one example, a study of the way seven national governments chose to adopt vaccines for pneumonia and diarrhoeal diseases found that decisions were sometimes guided by standard economic evaluations (cost-effectiveness analysis), but also by unanticipated derivatives of it: short-term costs; funding available from the Global Alliance on Vaccines and Immunization (GAVI); estimates of the burden of disease to be overcome; and local political priorities, among others (Chapter 2).

The form of the interaction between health providers and consumers (competitions, games, markets, nudges, wagers, and others), and the criteria for choice (premises of analysis), are themselves matters for investigation, and there have been too few investigations of this kind; a normative analysis that guesses these criteria a priori is in danger of producing the right answer to the wrong question.

Health accounts

Investment in prevention today, directly or indirectly, short- and long-term, is far greater than the 3% of global health spending suggested by the international System of Health Accounts (SHA). However, to assess the value of spending on prevention, we need to know how much greater, and with what results.

The SHA is an indispensable tool for tracking expenditure within health-care systems, following well-defined criteria (Box 2.2), but excludes expenditure in other sectors that have indirect effects on health. An analysis here of global trends in morbidity and mortality shows that about half of all deaths averted between 1990 and 2017 were due to the prevention of illness rather than to reductions in death following illness, including effects that operate outside the health sector (and outside the scope of the SHA; Chapter 2).

Despite their importance, there is no systematic method of counting investments in prevention beyond the SHA, or of assessing its full impact. There are, however, models to build on. One of these is Trackfin, a financial monitoring system for water, sanitation, and hygiene (WASH; Chapter 2). Trackfin has shown that many countries spend more on WASH, with its many benefits, than on all aspects of public health and prevention covered by the SHA.

Inclusive benefits

The total value of prevention is the sum of all the multiple benefits (all the hazards removed). Actions taken earlier (upstream) in the causal chain of illness usually have a wider range of effects, so the benefits (and the costs) should be measured with respect to particular interventions, rather than in terms of specific risks to health (downstream 'risk factors') or health conditions (hazards; Chapter 2).

Tuberculosis (TB) control illustrates the value of putting one disease in the wider context. There are many known 'risk factors' for TB. Almost all of them account, separately, for a small fraction of TB cases and deaths, but mitigating these risks has substantial additional benefits for health (diabetes, undernutrition) and society (homelessness, crowding; Chapter 5).

The full value of a sanitary system puts the costs and the health benefits (preventing infection and disease in environments contaminated with human and animal faeces) alongside those for agriculture (farm animal and crop productivity, excreta as fertilizer), education (girls attending school), energy production (biofuels), environmental protection (disposal of excreta and wastewater, water conservation), and infrastructure development (flood prevention, access paths, and roads). Together these amount to the total return on investment in sanitation, which is usually underestimated (Chapters 2 and 7).

Likewise, better health adds to the diverse benefits of climate change mitigation and adaptation. Health is protected through relief from the heat stress, air pollution, droughts, floods, storms, and wildfires that are linked to greenhouse gas (GHG) emissions. Health also benefits indirectly from improvements in nutrition (low-meat, plant-rich diets), transportation (lower vehicle emissions, active travel), air quality (low-emission stoves), energy supply (power from renewable sources), and waste management (improved water treatment; Chapter 8).

All three of these examples—TB control, improved sanitation, and action on climate change—show how human health contributes to, and profits from, healthy economies, environments, and societies, as framed by the 17 Sustainable Development Goals (SDGs; Chapter 8). The SDGs are a ready-made agenda for prevention, incorporating the numerous interconnections between health (SDG 3) and all the other factors affecting health and well-being (Chapter 3).

Across these interconnections, a vast array of causes and effects remains to be investigated, with the potential to reveal more options for prevention. As one example among many, new research is evaluating the full costs and benefits of transport policies, going beyond road injuries and air pollution, adding in other advantages such as increased physical activity (Chapter 6, and below). Inclusive accounting of this kind generates the evidence needed to put health, through prevention, in all government policies, and transport policies contribute to at least 12 of the 17 SDGs (Chapter 3).

Health accountability

Accountancy underpins accountability—the process of assigning liability and responsibility for illness or injury to causes and (in)actions.

Clinical, curative medicine is personal; prevention is typically nameless. A sick patient with an identity is intrinsically more important than an anonymous person who is yet to become ill. One corollary is that errors of commission (e.g. an inappropriate and harmful medical treatment) carry greater accountability than errors of omission (the failure to prevent illness, in individuals or populations; Chapter 2). One solution is to translate impersonal statistics—for example, about food shortages and malnutrition—into (representative) personal stories about hunger and starvation (Chapter 8).

Methods for tying effects to causes are central to epidemiology (what did it) and to the law (who did it), among other means of defining causality. 'Attribution science' is bringing the two together, though the strength of evidence required by epidemiology and the law may differ, as do the consequences of decisions made in each domain.

Cigarette smoking damages health and tobacco companies are being held legally responsible. Glyphosate weedkiller is 'probably carcinogenic to humans' (as a cause of non-Hodgkin's lymphoma); that attribution of hazard by the International Agency for Research on Cancer has underpinned successful litigation against its manufacturer in the United States. Going beyond the limits of causality in epidemiology, the legal judgment linked glyphosate exposure to cancer in a single individual. Climate change is causing more droughts, floods, hurricanes, and wildfires, and it is now possible to calculate the probability that a specific event was due to climate change: thus, human influence through GHG emissions was to blame for an estimated 75% of the elevated risk of death in Europe's 2003 heatwave. Thousands of cases of climate change litigation are now in process worldwide (Chapter 8).

Some preventable causes of harm are subject only to weaker forms of accountability. Between 2012 and 2017, UK government economic policies led to a period of austerity that probably caused hundreds of thousands of premature deaths. Epidemiologists concluded that a causal link is likely if not definite; economists differed over the need for policies that led to austerity in the first place. In the end, judgement about who is culpable, if anyone, is likely to rest with the electorate rather than with the judiciary (Chapter 3). Delayed government actions in response to the COVID-19 pandemic, leading to hundreds of thousands of preventable deaths, are another case in point.

Prevention as health promotion

The larger goal of prevention is to create better health and well-being, 'not merely the absence of disease or infirmity.'[2] The age-old adage could thus be extended: 'prevention is better than cure, but promotion is healthier for sure'. Just as incentives are needed to discourage harmful behaviours, they are needed to encourage healthy behaviours too.

In behavioural science, tests of 'prospect theory' have found that people tend to be loss-averse; they dislike losses (e.g. of money) more than equivalent gains, and they are more willing to take risks to avoid those losses. The circumstances under which prospect theory applies to gaining or losing health, and hence the value of health promotion or disease prevention, are still open to investigation (Chapter 2). It is clear, however, that the promotion of healthier lifestyles has a better chance of success when the enticements are strong: based on laws and regulations rather than guidelines and voluntary codes of conduct; and where the benefits for health are large, numerous, and complementary.

Legislation can promote healthy eating, as well as discouraging unhealthy eating, in a variety of ways: through lower sales taxes on fruits and vegetables, favourable leasing terms for grocery stores, and others. In addition, subsidies for healthy foods work as well as taxes on harmful foods, so long as the price changes are big enough (in the order of 10%–15%; Chapter 6).

Physical inactivity is notoriously immovable, but there are successful models. Offering multiple benefits, the low-cost, get-fit, sociable Parkrun scheme, launched in the UK in 2004, now takes place weekly in 22 countries worldwide (Chapter 6).

Mixing incentives and disincentives, deterrents to car use go hand in hand with the provision of convenient and safe walking and cycling paths in towns and cities. However, the promotion of active lifestyles for better health invariably has a wider context. Helsinki's successful active transportation programme—limiting car use in the city, and coupling public transport with easier ways to cycle and walk—was not driven primarily by health but by a vision of how the city could be made more liveable—aesthetically appealing, safe, and easy to get around. In Helsinki, as elsewhere, health has to make its claims among all other government priorities. Once again, this is the practical business of putting health in all policies (HiAP; Chapter 3)—of making health integral to well-being.

Hazards and perceptions

When future hazards are perceived to be greater threats, so are the benefits of preventing them. If perceptions and subjective values influence choices, they should be made explicit in the analysis of costs and benefits.

Behavioural science has compiled a long list of reasons why hazards and risks are perceived to be more and less important than their objectively measured values. Risks cause greater anxiety when imposed, uncontrollable, and unpredictable. Hazards are disproportionately threatening when novel, acute, dreaded, and man-made (Chapter 2). Familiar endemic diseases that change little from year to year, such as TB, parasitic worm infections, and childhood diarrhoeal diseases are rarely seen as health emergencies, even though they remain major causes of death around the world (Chapters 2, 5, and 7). Public fears of these diseases are allayed in part by an awareness of the options for prevention and treatment, but normality contributes to neglect.

One way to raise the profile of diseases as familiar as TB is to highlight new dangers from these old hazards, such as the emergence of multi-drug resistant strains, or the risk of resurgence when health services fail. Both resurgence and resistance changed the outlook on TB control in the US during the 1980s (the 'U-shaped curve of concern') and in former Soviet countries during the 1990s. In these instances, there were large, underestimated costs for lapses of TB control. Decades later, the recovery in both parts of the world is still incomplete (Chapter 5).

Optimizing prevention

Interventions in the causal chain of illness run along the spectrum from prevention (upstream) to cure (downstream). The case for prevention rests on finding ways to be more efficient upstream than downstream, delivering benefits that are large enough (effective), costs that are low enough (affordable), or both together (value for money).

The case studies in Chapters 3–8 explored the efficiency of prevention in a variety of settings; some examples are repeated in summary here: on financing health services, pandemic preparedness, TB and HIV/AIDS control, and climate change.

According to SHA data, a large fraction of the budgets for prevention and public health in Organisation for Economic Co-operation and Development countries is spent on health check-ups (healthy condition monitoring [HCM]), which are not generally considered to be cost-effective. One solution is to improve efficiency by targeting people at higher risk. Thus, in certain age groups, screening for early signs of breast, cervical, and colorectal cancers is usually cost-effective against standard benchmarks (Chapter 3).

The drawback of targeting is that effectiveness (total benefit) may be sacrificed for cost-effectiveness (value for money). The problem is greater when more of the illness in a population occurs among a large number of people, each of whom is at low risk. The tension is captured by Geoffrey Rose's 'paradox of prevention', which arises when 'a measure that brings large benefits to the community offers little to each participating individual' (Chapter 1).[3] In this context, HCM leans towards effectiveness, rather than cost-effectiveness, even though its impact is doubtful (Chapter 3).

Primary prevention applies to populations as well as individuals, but some methods of protecting populations are more efficient than others. Screening wild and domestic animals for a virus that might cause the next epidemic—the World Health Organization's Disease 'X'—is not generally efficient because the cross-over of zoonotic pathogens into human populations is unpredictable. There are alternative ways of preventing outbreaks of new infections: the regulation of trade in wildlife and bush meat, and the control of deforestation where humans contact animal sources of infection. However, primary prevention always needs a back-up: systems for surveillance, early detection, and rapid response (secondary prevention) have a vital and proven role in containing disease outbreaks in their early stages, whatever the emerging pathogen (Chapter 4).

The spread of COVID-19 across the world in 2020 regenerated the argument that there should be no trade-off between health and the economy. On the scale of whole nations, countries with swifter and more forceful responses to COVID-19 reported fewer deaths and smaller economic losses, protecting both lives and livelihoods. In some countries, the costs of intervening early were probably less than the benefits (i.e. the averted costs of not intervening). But delayed intervention presented plenty of difficult and costly choices in the countries worst affected by COVID-19: between school closures and the imperative for education; between border restrictions to keep out infection and the need to maintain tourism and trade.

COVID-19 is unlikely to be eradicated globally, though it can be eliminated temporarily and locally, as shown by Australia and New Zealand, among other countries. From 2021 onwards, the challenge worldwide is to keep the disease at low levels by means other than costly lockdowns of society. There are now better ways to prevent infection and illness, led by vaccination for all, backed by improved diagnostics for efficient testing (with isolation) and contact tracing (with quarantine) during local outbreaks, and supported by improved curative treatments.

For communicable diseases where patients are infectious and ill at the same time, and for which there are curative drugs, there is no dilemma in the choice between prevention and cure: drugs kill the pathogen and neutralize infectiousness at the same time. For both HIV/AIDS and TB, 'treatment as prevention', with antiviral and antibacterial drugs respectively, halts life-threatening illness and stops the transmission of infection (Chapter 5).

The principal goal of climate change mitigation is to end GHG emissions (primary prevention), but adaptation (secondary prevention) is the essential back-up when mitigation fails. Adaptation is inferior to mitigation in the sense that action is remedial rather than preventive. But adaptation has efficiency in its favour: there are strong incentives for local adaptation to counter specific and probable local threats, such as extreme urban temperatures, flooding, and water scarcity. Responding to these threats is imperative, is often under autonomous local control, and gives predictable returns on investment. Furthermore, action does not depend on making the causal link between, for example, flooding and GHG emissions (Chapter 8).

Risk and insurance

Almost all potential hazards are manageable, provided the cost is commensurate with the avoidable risk. To satisfy that criterion, a general tactic is to pool the risks and share the costs. This is health insurance to preserve health, rather than to cover the cost of treating illness.

For single, major causes of illness and premature death, each risk is worth confronting directly, and this is being done with varying degrees of success: indoor air pollution more quickly than ambient outdoor air pollution, tobacco more quickly than illicit drugs (Chapter 6). In contrast to the many small risks for TB ('Inclusive benefits' above), co-infection with HIV and *Mycobacterium tuberculosis* greatly increases the chance of developing TB disease. Consequently, antiretroviral treatment (ART) to suppress HIV infection has prevented millions of cases of TB, especially in sub-Saharan Africa, adding to the large and direct benefits of ART for patients and populations affected by HIV/AIDS (Chapter 5).

The instruments of insurance are more relevant in preparedness for epidemics, pandemics, and other unlikely disasters. Most of these threats are low-risk hazards with uncertain timing and potentially large impact. Insurance works by pooling the risks (so that the total avoidable risk is bigger and more predictable) and sharing the costs (so that the cost per person is lower). There are various imaginative ways of insuring against emergencies. Some of these are: invest in preparedness for multiple rather than single pathogens (early detection and response systems); expand the number of people who are willing to share the cost by including everyone who might be exposed (risk of HIV/AIDS); coordinate investment in generic platforms for the rapid development of new technologies against multiple pathogens (vaccine development); reinforce incentives for international collaboration under the International Health Regulations (IHR 2005); expand data-sharing mechanisms as a basis for collective action (databases for pathogen genomes); and exploit the different but complementary strengths of multiple organizations (Chapter 4).

The inevitable competition for scarce resources suggests one further tactic: invest in preparedness during 'peace time': before an emergency demands extra resources for medical care. During a cholera outbreak, for instance, the priority is to detect and treat cases early, reinforce surveillance, monitor the safety of water sources, and organize a vaccination campaign. Investment in a water and sanitation system usually has to wait (Chapters 2 and 7).

Valuing the future, today

Faced with an impending threat, the willingness to act promptly depends on how the threat is valued today. One way to assign value to a future loss (or gain) is to put a price on it.

Excise taxes, on tobacco or gasoline, for example, present consumers and manufacturers with choices, calibrated by governments. Consumers can pay a higher price today for the costs incurred to society in future; or they can save the money and adopt tobacco-free and non-polluting lifestyles. Manufacturers must decide whether and how to continue producing tobacco and gasoline with reduced sales. Governments benefit from tax revenues so long as the goods continue to be bought and sold, but politicians generally need more than revenue to defend the imposition of taxes against opposition. Consequently, tobacco and gasoline, like sugar-sweetened foods and drinks, are usually under-taxed: their prices do not reflect the full costs to citizens or society. Gasoline illustrates the more general problem of taxing carbon to cut GHG emissions. The current price of carbon is currently too low; it may rise, but carbon taxes anyway need to be reinforced by other incentives, including subsidies for wind, solar, hydrogen, and hydropower (Chapters 6 and 8).

Because the power, industrial, and transport sectors still depend heavily on fossil fuels, the world is far from a trajectory that will prevent the global temperature from rising more than 2°C above pre-industrial levels, as stipulated by the 2015 Paris Agreement. And yet there are reasons to be hopeful about action on climate change. Tipping points in the climate system threaten to drive abrupt, irreversible changes to physical and ecological systems—deserts, forests, ice sheets, and ocean currents. But there are likely to be thresholds in the social response system too: pushing at 'sensitive intervention points' could trigger sudden shifts away from investment in fossil fuels, accelerating progress towards cleaner energy. Questions about how to engineer such rapid changes in practice, and about the role of health as a catalyst, are being answered by the mix of more (e.g. Brazil, Canada, Chile) and less (e.g. France) successful experiences to date (Chapter 8).

Cooperation and collective action

Taxes (and regulations) are not merely devices for valuing the future, or for providing governments with income: they are also a means of stimulating cooperation and collective action. Collective action is not exclusive to prevention, but most preventive methods depend on it.

Taxes on the production and consumption of harmful products are sometimes seen as punishment ('sin taxes'), or the cosseting interference of a 'nanny state'. More positively, taxation is a part of the social contract between consumers in pursuit of healthier lifestyles and governments that, besides satisfying a duty of care, earn revenue by supporting that goal; for 'the end of law is not to abolish or restrain, but to preserve and enlarge freedom' (Chapter 6).[4]

The 2020 UK strategy to tackle obesity recognizes that dietary choices are not the responsibility of individual consumers alone, but also depend on the choices on offer and the circumstances that shape those choices. If individuals or families are trying to switch to a healthy diet, they must be able to buy fresh foods locally at an affordable price. But, even when these are available, many still want help to make healthy choices in the face of commercial forces and personal preferences for sugary and salty foods. General guidelines for voluntary action are generally ignored; legislation and regulation are more effective, including obligatory calorie labelling in restaurants and cafes, plus the prohibition of TV advertising to children of foods high in sugar or salt (Chapter 6).

When there are no fundamental conflicts of interest, or overwhelming commercial pressures, motives can sometimes be aligned through 'co-production'. In villages, communes, and neighbourhoods around the world, sanitary systems have been built on local preferences for toilets, sewage, and water-recycling systems. The bigger challenge, for sanitation as for other development initiatives, is to scale up from small communities to large municipalities and whole countries, where the spirit of co-production is hard to maintain. As demonstrated by Malaysia, Singapore, the Republic of Korea, and Thailand in their early years as nation states, sanitation at country scale needs a country-wide strategy, strong leadership, and determined implementation. Leadership creates a common vision of the future that gives context to, instead of being driven by, budgets, risks, hazards, and discount rates. The virtues of visionary leadership are, however, more easily described than replicated: the creation of sanitation systems, national health services and infectious disease control programmes (e.g. HIV/AIDS) invariably depends on historical and cultural contingencies (Chapters 3, 5, and 7).

Pathways to prevention

When the potential benefits of prevention are clear, it must also be clear how practically to achieve them.

Most current cases of lung cancer worldwide could have been prevented by not smoking cigarettes. Tobacco control measures increase prices through taxation, through bans on advertising, and by providing information about the harms of smoking. But all these measures are necessarily additional to the clinical treatment of lung cancer and other diseases caused by tobacco (Chapter 6). Medical treatment is the default. The practical implication for health services is that, even if economic evaluation favours prevention over cure, a programme of prevention requires additional, ring-fenced funding (within the scope of the SHA; Chapter 3). Shifting the balance towards prevention is a process of transition during which prevention, public health, and medicine coexist over years.

This example points to a weakness in much public health guidance: we are told the desired endpoint and, ideally, a reason for choosing it—an affordable, beneficial, or socially acceptable solution—but not how to get there. A ring-fenced budget for 'prevention and public health' (as defined by the SHA) is one pragmatic solution. The 2030 Agenda for Sustainable Development describes a few more: among the SDGs are selected 'means of implementation', including mechanisms for financing, technological innovation, developing skills, and creating partnerships.[5] But these are no more than helpful examples. To escape the health dilemma, we need a more detailed map—to navigate away from reactive medical treatment, bypassing illness and injury, on the road to a 'state of complete physical, mental, and social well-being'.[2]

Expanding the choices

Clearly, prevention is more likely to be feasible when there are more options to choose from. Every discipline calls for more money to support research and discovery, but underfunded prevention can make a special case.

For instance, TB control focuses on drug treatment, and so too does investment in research and development (R&D), ahead of vaccine and operational research (Chapter 5). Similarly, policies for cancer care have been supported by relatively few economic evaluations of preventive methods compared with disease detection and treatment (Chapter 6). The disinclination to fund prevention research might reflect the lack of commercial interest. However, new public and private partnerships to combat epidemics are showing how to create incentives for prevention—by sharing the risks and costs of R&D for diagnostics, vaccines, and other technologies (Chapter 4).

But the new options for prevention are not only technologies: there are novel financial and managerial tools as well. Some recent innovative ideas, such as the World Bank's Pandemic Emerging Finance Facility, have failed when put to the test. Others, including Development (DIBs) and Social Impact Bonds (SIBs) have as-yet unrealized potential; the principles are well-defined, but DIBs and SIBs have not yet become mainstream practice. More successfully, the World Bank's mechanism for linking funding to programme results has supported prevention in other ways—for example, by strengthening health, water, and sanitation systems around the world (Chapter 4).

Considering all the factors that might favour or disfavour prevention—the avoidable hazards and risks, the options and their costs—the case studies in Chapters 3–8 leave plenty of unanswered questions for research: What arguments will persuade governments to increase budgets for prevention and public health? How is cooperation best organized to prevent pandemics? How do cigarette smokers trade current pleasures against the risks and hazards of future illness? What are the most effective ways of promoting healthy diets and discouraging unhealthy ones? Will the argument for better health—made by epidemiology, economics, or in law—stimulate divestment from fossil fuels and towards investment in renewable energy?

The subtitle of this book poses the overarching question: is prevention better than cure? In principle, that depends on the costs and benefits of each option. In practice, prevention has had far more positive effects on health than portrayed by public health accounts—over recent years, and over preceding decades and centuries. In future, the benefits of prevention could be greater still. The 12 lessons of this concluding chapter are just a few of the ways to gain those greater rewards.

Summary

The argument in this book rests on a simple proposition: understanding the reason why people prefer to take a chance on sickness and cure is the key to persuading them when and why they should choose prevention instead. This final chapter summarizes the means of persuasion: investigate rather than presuppose which criteria are used to make health choices; build systems for accounting (inclusive costs and benefits of prevention) and for accountability (liability and responsibility); offer ways to improve health, not merely ways to avoid losing it; evaluate, in order to manage, the perceptions linked to health hazards; exploit the logic of choice to insure against the risk of unlikely disasters, to increase the present value of future threats, to foster cooperation as a basis for prevention, to map out the practical pathways to prevention, and to remedy the under-investment in prevention research. The tools of prevention are the means to a greater end—health as a 'state of complete physical, mental and social well-being'.

References

1. Fineberg HV. The paradox of disease prevention: Celebrated in principle, resisted in practice. *Journal of the American Medical Association* 2013; *310*: 85–90.
2. World Health Organization. *Constitution of the World Health Organization.* Geneva: World Health Organization; 2006.
3. Rose G. Strategy of prevention: Lessons from cardiovascular disease. *British Medical Journal (Clinical Research Edition)* 1981; *282*: 1847–51.

4. Locke J. *Two Treatises of Government (1821 edition)*. London: Whitmore and Fenn; 1689.

5. United Nations. Transforming our world: the 2030 Agenda for Sustainable Development. https://sustainabledevelopment.un.org/post2015/transforming-ourworld (accessed 7 January 2021).

Epilogue
Collective action for health

Once a year, Geneva's cycling enthusiasts get together for the Cyclotour du Léman, a 180-km bike race around the lake. In 2020, COVID-19 intervened, forcing postponement from warm May to cool October. Then, at the last minute, they restricted the route out of Geneva to a 55-km leg to Lausanne.

Some competitors sign up as a team. That's the sociable way to do it. It is faster too. Most amateur cyclists who are reasonably fit can maintain 25 km/h on their own for a few hours, but they can do 35 km/h or more when working as a team. 'Drafting' saves energy, so everyone can go faster while doing the same amount of work.

But a few competitors do sign up as singletons; sometimes they find soulmates on the road, sometimes not. This year I was not part of any team, so I went solo.

The start of the Cyclotour is always messy—a haphazard mix of fast and slow, of coalescing and disbanding groups, of risky manoeuvres at close quarters and high speed.

By Coppet (10 km), the fastest had got away from me, and the slowest were well behind. We converged to a bunch of five. Peloton etiquette began to take shape: every few minutes one group member took the lead, pushing the bow wave, while the rest took a breather in the slipstream.

By Gland (20 km), we were down to three, travelling at a sustainable if slightly quickish pace. Three is too few to be aerodynamically super-efficient, but the rhythm was stabilizing. Yellow (the colour of his waterproof) was riding Canyon Endurance, like me. Red (his Swiss flag emblem) I judged to be in my (older) age bracket. We both had about 30 years on Yellow. Now in our threesome, the front man no longer glanced back; he knew the other two would be right on the shoulder.

We adopted the usual leader's hand signals as alerts to small changes of direction and speed: hands downwards left or right to warn of potholes, grates, and kerbs; a finger twirl for an upcoming roundabout. But there was no signalling to indicate who should lead and when, apart from the general rule to take turns.

On good roads, the tyres on the Canyon are pumped to high pressure so the bike flies across the tarmac. The penalty is a harder ride: after 30 km, I picked up a back twinge, and handlebar numbness started to set in. Approaching the hill to Allaman (35 km), I stood up on the pedals for momentary relief. Yellow took the cue and moved into the lead. At Saint-Prex (40 km), I had a little more juice than the pace set by Red and pushed ahead.

From the halfway mark onwards, our unspoken compact meant that, barring accidents, we would finish together. The Cyclotour is billed as a race, but the winner of this one was of no consequence. In the event, Red nosed the chequered flag in Lausanne on 1h 47.33m, averaging 31 km/h. Not Tour de France pace, but we had raised our game as a team. Braking to a halt over the finish line, there was first eye contact among strangers and a brief exchange of smiles. A fist bump with Yellow. A thumbs up with Red. I didn't ask their names. They didn't ask mine. They didn't ask each other.

I picked up my 'refuelling' bag at the catering tent. A few metres ahead, late-morning sunlight skimmed off the still surface of the lake. Behind me, rain clouds were amassing over the Jura mountains where I live. I gulped down the Evian, ate the sandwich, and saved the Swiss chocolate for the slow ride back home.

Index

For the benefit of digital users, indexed terms that span two pages (e.g., 52–53) may, on occasion, appear on only one of those pages.

Tables, figures and boxes are indicated by *t*, *f* and *b* following the page number